D1548667

CANCER
Nursing Research
A Practical Approach

Marcia M. Grant, RN, DNSc, OCN
Director, Nursing Research and Education
City of Hope National Medical Center
Duarte, California

Geraldine V. Padilla, PhD
Associate Dean, Research
School of Nursing
University of California, Los Angeles
Los Angeles, California

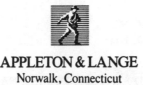

APPLETON & LANGE
Norwalk, Connecticut

0-8385-1033-7

Copyright © 1990 by Appleton & Lange
A Publishing Division of Prentice Hall

90 91 92 93 94 / 10 9 8 7 6 5 4 3 2 1

Prentice Hall International (UK) Limited, *London*
Prentice Hall of Australia Pty. Limited, *Sydney*
Prentice Hall Canada, Inc., *Toronto*
Prentice Hall Hispanoamericana, S.A., *Mexico*
Prentice Hall of India Private Limited, *New Delhi*
Prentice Hall of Japan, Inc., *Tokyo*
Simon & Schuster Asia Pte. Ltd., *Singapore*
Editora Prentice Hall do Brasil Ltda., *Rio de Janeiro*
Prentice Hall, *Englewood Cliffs, New Jersey*

Library of Congress Cataloging-in-Publication Data

Cancer nursing research: a practical approach/[edited by] Marcia M.
  Grant, Geraldine V. Padilla.
      p.   cm.
  Includes index.
  ISBN 0-8385-1033-7
  1. Cancer—Nursing—Research.   I. Grant, Marcia Moeller.
II. Padilla, Geraldine V.
  [DNLM: 1. Nursing Research—methods.   2. Oncologic Nursing.   WY
156 C21974]
RC266.C3563   1990
610.73'698'072—dc20
DNLM/DLC
for Library of Congress   89-15115
                                                                        CIP

Acquisitions Editor: Marion K. Welch
Production Editor: Amanda D. Egan
Designer: Janice Barsevich

PRINTED IN THE UNITED STATES OF AMERICA

This book is dedicated to the patients who have participated in cancer nursing studies and to the many nurses and students who have sharpened our research efforts.

Reviewers

Nancy Bergstrom, RN, PhD
Professor
College of Nursing
University of Nebraska Medical Center
Omaha, Nebraska

Marilyn Frank-Stromborg, RN, EdD, FAAN
Professor
School of Nursing
Northern Illinois University
DeKalb, Illinois

Kathryn Graham, PhD, RN, FAAN
Professor and Chair, Community Care Systems
School of Nursing
University of Washington
Seattle, Washington

Darlene W. Mood, PhD
Associate Professor
College of Nursing
Wayne State University
Detroit, Michigan

Madeline H. Schmitt, RN, PhD
Associate Professor
School of Nursing
University of Rochester
Rochester, New York

Ora L. Strickland, PhD, RN, FAAN
Professor, Doctoral Program
School of Nursing
University of Maryland at Baltimore
Baltimore, Maryland

Contributors

Paula Anderson, RN, MN
Project Director
Department of Nursing Research and Education
City of Hope National Medical Center
Duarte, California

Jan Atwood, RN, PhD, FAAN
Professor, College of Nursing
Behavioral Sciences Coordinator
Cancer Prevention and Control, Cancer Center
University of Arizona
Tucson, Arizona

Marylin J. Dodd, RN, PhD
Associate Professor
Department of Physiological Nursing
University of California, San Francisco
San Francisco, California

Marcia M. Grant, RN, DNSc, OCN
Director, Nursing Research and Education
City of Hope National Medical Center
Duarte, California

Mel R. Haberman, RN, PhD
Director of Clinical Nursing Research
Fred Hutchinson Cancer Research Center
Seattle, Washington

Robert Hill, PhD
Assistant Director
Department of Biostatistics
City of Hope National Medical Center
Duarte, California

Frances Marcus Lewis, RN, PhD
Professor
School of Nursing
University of Washington
Seattle, Washington

Ruth McCorkle, RN, PhD, FAAN
Professor
School of Nursing
University of Pennsylvania
Philadelphia, Pennsylvania

Gerald Metter, PhD[†]
Formerly Director
Department of Biostatistics
City of Hope National Medical Center
Duarte, California

Geraldine V. Padilla, PhD
Associate Dean, Research
School of Nursing
University of California, Los Angeles
Los Angeles, California

Eleanor Saltzer, RN, PhD, FAAN
Consultant
Research and Practice
Orange, California

[†]Deceased

Contents

Preface

The purpose of this book is threefold: to provide beginning nurse investigators with a practical guide for the research process; to provide research faculty with a teaching tool including specific examples for steps in the research process; and to provide both beginning and experienced investigators with information to help implement studies in clinical settings.

The book augments information in basic research textbooks. It is written from the viewpoint of experienced investigators who have carried out a variety of oncology nursing studies in clinical settings, have taught research in university and clinical settings, have served on scientific nursing and cancer review committees responsible for judging the worthiness of research applications for funding, and have served on human subjects review committees responsible for approving research proposals. Thus, the book reflects the collective, practical experience of scientists who understand what it takes to develop a valid, feasible, cancer nursing study.

The book addresses key issues in cancer nursing research beginning with the expansion of research in this nursing specialty. In Chapter 2, discussion of progress in cancer nursing research provides the types of questions studied in the past and needing future investigation. The information on the development of the research question provided in Chapter 3 helps the reader formulate questions emerging from clinical insights and theoretical perspectives. Chapter 4 discusses some theoretical frameworks that are relevant to cancer nursing research and their formulation and importance. Criteria to consider in selecting the appropriate experimental, quasi-experimental, or descriptive research design are explained in Chapter 5, as are the limitations of these designs. Chapter 6 presents the issues that are relevant to research data and ties together the research question, design, and methodology in relation to the reliability and validity of research variables. Chapter 7 introduces the basic statistical principles and methods used in cancer nursing research with emphasis on both the logic and the level of uncertainty underlying the inferential process. Because the ability to critique research reports is important in evaluating the applicability of findings to future studies or clinical practice, the basic criteria used to judge the value of study findings is discussed in Chapter 8. Finally, practical strategies for managing projects are explained in Chapters 9 and 10. These strategies cover important topics such as obtaining support from colleagues, other disciplines, and administration; identifying sources of financial support; training of research assistants; developing data manuals; and administering budgets.

At the end of the text, summaries of seven research articles serve as examples of different kinds of cancer nursing studies. These studies are discussed throughout the various chapters to illustrate different aspects of the research process and offer continuity across the chapters. The book is organized along the lines of the research process. Some overlap between chapters is necessary so that each chapter can stand alone.

We would like to acknowledge the support of Stuart Horton, formerly of Appleton & Lange, as well as our present editor, Janet Walsh Foltin. We would also like to thank our contributing authors. Each one of them is a well-known, experienced cancer nursing researcher whose daily work has provided the means to make this a practical book. We believe by sharing their knowledge and recommendations, the work of research will be made easier for others.

Marcia M. Grant, RN, DNSc, OCN
Geraldine V. Padilla, PhD

CHAPTER 1

Research: An Expanding Component of the Cancer Nursing Specialty

Marcia M. Grant

The recent and rapid development of cancer nursing research provides evidence that research is an expanding component of this nursing specialty (Padilla & Grant, 1987). This development appears to be related to a number of factors: the characteristics of the nurses who practice this specialty, the characteristics of the environment in which cancer patients are cared for, and increasing professional activities that include research as a focus.

CHARACTERISTICS OF ONCOLOGY NURSES

In 1989, the Oncology Nursing Society (ONS) reported a membership of 15,198 members, of whom 14,647 were active RNs (Kinzler, 1989). Established in 1975 as the specialty organization for nurses caring for cancer patients, ONS has grown steadily. The 1989 membership represents an increase of 2578 members during 1988. Licensed registered nurses in the United States number 2.1 million, with 80 percent or 1.2 million actively employed either full-time or part-time (Aiken & Mullinix, 1987). Members of the ONS represent less than 1 percent of this total nursing population. However, ONS is not atypical when sizes of other nursing specialty organizations are compared. ONS falls in the middle size range, with the operating room nursing and the critical care nursing groups being the largest organizations and groups such as the pediatric oncology nurses being considerably smaller ones. Information about ONS members is the principal source of available information about characteristics of nurses who care for cancer patients.

Two surveys provide evidence of the research interests and involvement of the members of the oncology nursing specialty organization. Grant and Stromborg (1981) reported findings of a survey conducted by the ONS Research Committee. This survey was mailed to the total 1980 membership of ONS (N = 2205) and was returned by 988 members, indicating a response rate of 45 percent. The respondents reported a high degree of interest in participating in research, with 42 percent giving research a large or highest priority, 41 percent giving it a moderate priority, and 17 percent giving it a lower or no priority. A majority of the respondents (52 percent) had participated in research as part of their educational experiences, 40 percent reported participating in one to three projects after completion of their last educational experience. Participation involved a variety of tasks associated with research implementation. Data collection was by far the most common activity, with 75 percent of the respondents reporting this as part of their nursing role. Clinical protocol implementation was done by 42 percent, data analysis by 37 percent, writing up project results by 36 percent, and developing a research protocol by 35 percent. A reported 10 percent (N = 95) of the respondents had published research results.

The level of education reported by the nurses in ONS attests to the potential for participating in research. A comparison of the educational preparation of the members of the American Nurses' Association with that of members of the ONS revealed a higher percentage of nurses with baccalaureate preparation (39 percent versus 25 percent) and with master preparation (24 percent versus 16 percent) (Grant & Stromborg, 1981). Considering this level of education, one could expect the average oncology nurse to have a beginning understanding and interest in research.

Some changes in the characteristics of oncology nurses were revealed in the second survey (McGuire, Frank–Stromborg, & Varricchio, 1985). Participants in this survey responded to a questionnaire published in the *Oncology Nursing Forum,* which requested the readership to complete and return it. Only 350 members responded representing a considerably smaller percentage of the total membership than the first time. However, respondents were from 46 states; thus they represented a broad geographic area. The typical respondent (1) had either a baccalaureate or master's degree; (2) had been in nursing under ten years and in oncology nursing less than six years; (3) worked in a hospital setting or a school of nursing; and (4) was employed as either a clinical specialist or an educator. A major difference reported in the 1984 survey was the increase in the number and variety of research roles in which participation was identified. In the 1981 survey, the primary role reported was that of a data collector (75 percent), whereas in 1984, respondents were involved predominantly in nurse-directed research and in a variety of activities including literature search, proposal development, individual investigation, statistical analysis, in addition to data collection. These expanding roles in research reflect expanding sophistication and general involvement in research by oncology nurses in clinical and educational settings.

CHARACTERISTICS OF THE ENVIRONMENT

Another factor important in oncology nurses' expanding role in the conduct of nursing research is the environment in which cancer patients are cared for, because it is one rich in research questions and opportunities. After the enactment of the National Cancer Act in 1971, federal funding was made available to combat cancer. Federal funding for the development of cancer centers throughout the United States resulted in the rapid implementation of clinical trials of cancer treatment methods. The National Cancer Act supported the rapid dissemination of results of these trials from the large teaching centers where most of the research was conducted to the communities where most cancer patients were being treated (Clive & Mortenson, 1988). In 1974 the formation of the Association of Community Cancer Centers, also funded by the National Cancer Act, provided support for establishment of the same kind of clinical environment and resources in the community as was available at the cancer centers. Today, one out of every four cancer patients cared for in the United States is treated at one of these community cancer centers (Mortenson & Ney, 1988).

The development of cancer centers and community cancer centers becomes important in relation to the proportion of cancer patients that participate in medical research. Clinical research, more commonly called clinical trials, is one of the primary functions of the cancer centers that is now carried out by community cancer centers as well. Since 85 percent of the cancer patients are cared for in the community as opposed to the cancer centers, the development of community cancer centers provided access to clinical trials for a large proportion of cancer patients. In fact, in 1987 approximately 50 percent of all new patients entered onto National Cancer Institute clinical research protocols were accrued from community cancer centers (Mortenson & Ney, 1988). Thus, a large proportion of cancer patients being cared for both in cancer centers located in large teaching institutions and in community hospitals that are members of the community cancer centers are participating in clinical trials of medical treatment. Each of these patients has a nurse who is helping to accrue data for research and who may be involved in a variety of ways in nursing research trials.

Clinical trial participation generally occurs through affiliation with the National Cooperative Research Groups, such as the Radiation Oncology Treatment Group (RTOG), the National Surgical Adjuvant Breast and Bowel Project (NSABP), and the Southwestern Oncology Group (SWOG) (Mortenson & Ney, 1988). Within each of these cooperative groups, nursing subcommittees are responsible for the implementation of medical clinical trials. In some of these committees, nursing protocols have been developed as well and implemented across a variety of institutions. For example, the Northern California Oncology

Group Nursing Subcommittee has a current clinical protocol for care of extravasations occurring from administration of chemotherapy. An additional mechanism available for nursing research is piggybacking a nursing research question onto an existing medical protocol. An example of such an arrangement is the adding of quality-of-life measurements to a medical protocol comparing surgical and radiation treatment of breast cancer.

The organization of cancer care has been shaped by funding from the National Cancer Institute, and this has resulted in a large proportion of cancer patients participating in clinical research. In addition, the nurses caring for these patients are exposed to the implementation of clinical trials, and for some of them, clinical nursing research.

Besides the rich background for research provided by the environment in which cancer patients are cared for, the nature of the disease and treatment result in biopsychosocial problems with accompanying questions related to clinical nursing care. For example, immunosuppression is common and can produce life-threatening infections and bleeding disorders, both of which are clinical problems that provide challenging nursing research problems. Radical surgical procedures can produce major changes in body image, which is also a nursing research interest. Daily radiation therapy can quickly drain family resources to pay for transportation and home-care support. Rapid development of new high-tech equipment shapes the nature of clinical nursing care and how it is delivered. Products to be evaluated include new pumps for feeding patients, for delivering intravenous medications, and new devices to prevent alopecia. Patient-administered analgesic devices and earlier discharge approaches prompt nurses to teach patients self-care for interventions usually controlled by the nurse. Do patients learn this self-care adequately? Are the rates of complications with these new methods within acceptable limits? Is the family able to cope with these changes? Do the changes impact on the patient's quality of life? Questions for study are abundant.

Recent changes in settings in which cancer patients are cared for has led to the development of new research questions for nurses. Cancer used to be a disease of hospitalized patients. Now patients are cared for in ambulatory settings and in the home (Brown, 1985). Nursing care is delivered in all these settings, and major challenges to nurses occur in efforts to coordinate the care between settings. In fact, the current nursing shortage reflects the need for nurses in these additional settings (Aiken & Mullinix, 1987). Questions that have resulted concern how high-tech care is delivered safely in the home, how communication about nursing problems is accomplished between the hospital nurse and the home-care nurse, and how patients are taught to carry out procedures involving sophisticated equipment and complicated procedures. Several major nursing studies are currently being conducted on issues surrounding home care for cancer patients (Given, 1987–1989, Padilla, 1986–1989, McCorkle, 1987–1990). Results of these and other studies will be needed to begin to understand and resolve the current problems in the provision of nursing care for cancer patients.

In summary, environmental characteristics have influenced the inclusion of research in the current role of the oncology nurse. These characteristics include the frequency with which cancer patients participate in medical research, the nature of the disease and the treatment, and the changes in settings used to care for cancer patients.

PROFESSIONAL ACTIVITIES

As well as the characteristics of the oncology nurse and the oncology environment, a variety of professional activities have influenced the expansion of the research role for the oncology nurse. The establishment of a clinical nursing research position in a clinical cancer center occurred in 1969 (Ayers, 1972). This position still exists and has been a rich source of nursing studies (Grant, 1989). Graduate programs for oncology nursing are growing, with 44 master's programs and one doctoral program reported in 1988 (McGee, 1988). Funding sources to support nursing research have expanded as well (*see* Chapter 9).

An additional impetus to the expansion of the research role for oncology nurses is the establishment of a Short Course for Oncology Nurses, a one-day workshop sponsored by the Oncology Nursing Society and the National Cancer Institute. Begun in 1984, this annual course is intended to prepare increased numbers of nurses to conduct studies relevant to influencing the care of individuals with cancer and their families (Grant, 1989). Ten students, either post master's, predoctoral, or postdoctoral, are selected anonymously from self-submitted research abstracts each year. The course includes student presentations of a proposed or ongoing study, which are followed by critiques of the research by two of four expert oncology faculty, who are selected on the basis of their experience in oncology research and graduate education. From 1984 to 1989, 99 post-master's students, 37 doctoral students, and 14 postdoctoral students have participated. Course participants from 1984 to 1986 have published 14 papers related to their presented research and submitted 34 grant proposals, of which 27 were funded. Clearly, this course has made a substantial impact on research conducted by oncology nurses.

A different perspective on professional activities influencing oncology nursing research appears when the nature of the research being conducted by the discipline as a whole is examined as well as that by individual researchers. When examined as a whole, nursing research related to cancer patients has increased to the point where clusters of studies in the same area are now available (Lindsey, 1985a, 1985b). Such clusters include studies concerned with alleviation of nausea and vomiting associated with chemotherapy and with breast self-examination. Analysis of such clusters make it possible to compare findings across studies, conduct replications when indicated, and accumulate evidence about the scientific foundations for cancer nursing practice. Use of cluster findings in clinical practice increases the scientific basis for clinical nursing care.

Further evidence of professional activities is seen when the nature of research activities by specific investigators across a span of years is examined. Programs of research are evident. Examples of these programs include the studies on self-care of cancer patients conducted by Dodd (1982, 1984), on the impact of cancer on the family conducted by Lewis, Ellison, and Woods (1985) and Stetz, Lewis, and Primomo (1986), and on quality of life of cancer patients conducted by Padilla, et al (1983), Grant, et al (1984), and Padilla and Grant (1985).

SUMMARY

In summary, a number of factors appear to be involved in the recent and rapid development of cancer nursing research. Specifically, characteristics of today's oncology nurses, the nature of the environment in which patients are cared for, and recent professional activities give evidence of an increase in interest, educational preparation, and research training. Examination of some of the studies being conducted shows trends toward clusters of studies by groups of investigators and programs of research conducted by single investigators. These facts illustrate the growth of oncology nursing as a scientifically based clinical discipline. Research is an acceptable and expected activity in many cancer nursing settings.

REFERENCES

Aiken, L.H., & Mullinix, C.F. (1987). The nurse shortage: Myth or reality? *The New England Journal of Medicine, 317*(10), 641–646.

Ayers, R. (1972). *Nursing service in transition.* Duarte, CA: City of Hope Medical Center.

Brown, J.K. (1985). Ambulatory services: The mainstay of cancer nursing care. *Oncology Nursing Forum, 12*(1), 57–59.

Clive, R.E., & Mortenson, L. E. (1988). Leadership in quality cancer care: The association of community cancer centers. In L. E. Mortenson (Ed.), *Community cancer programs in the United States: 1987–88.* Rockville, MD: Association of Community Cancer Centers.

Dodd, M.J. (1982). Cancer patients' knowledge of chemotherapy: Assessment and informational interventions. *Oncology Nursing Forum, 9*(3), 39–44.

Dodd, M.J. (1984). Patterns of self-care in cancer patients receiving radiation therapy. *Oncology Nursing Forum, 11*(3), 23–27.

Given, B. (1987–1989). Family homecare for cancer community-based model. Unpublished nursing research grant NR01915, National Center for Nursing Research, National Institutes of Health.

Grant, M.M., Padilla, G.V., Presant, C. et al. (1984). Cancer patients and quality of life. *Proceedings of the Fourth National Conference on Cancer Nursing.* New York: American Cancer Society.

Grant, M.M., & Stromborg, M. (1981). Promoting research collaboration: ONS research committee survey. *Oncology Nursing Forum, 8*(2), 48–53.

Grant, M.M. (1989). Department of Nursing Research and Education Annual Report, Duarte, CA: City of Hope National Medical Center.

Kinzler, J. (Personal Communication, June 13, 1989).

Lewis, F.M., Ellison, E.S., Woods, N.F. (1985). The impact of breast cancer on the family. *Seminars in Oncology Nursing, 1*(3), 206–213.

Lindsey, A.M. (1985a). Building the knowledge base for practice, part I: Nausea and vomiting. *Oncology Nursing Forum, 12*(1), 49–56.

Lindsey, A.M. (1985b). Building the knowledge base for practice, part II. Alopecia, breast self-exam and other human responses. *Oncology Nursing Forum, 12*(2), 27–34.

McCorkle, R. (1987–1990). Evaluation of home care for cancer patients. Unpublished nursing research grant NR01914, National Center for Nursing Research, Institutes of Health.

McGee, R. (1988). Survey of graduate programs in cancer nursing. *Oncology Nursing Forum, 15*(1), 90–96.

McGuire, D., Frank–Stromborg, M., Varricchio, C. (1985). 1984 ONS research committee survey of membership's research interest and involvement. *Oncology Nursing Forum, 12*(2), 99–103.

Mortenson, L.E., & Ney, M.S. (1988). Standards of quality and hospital cancer program characteristics. In L.E. Mortenson, (Ed.), *Community cancer programs in the United States: 1987–88,* Rockville, MD: Association of Community Cancer Centers.

Padilla, G.F. (1986–1990). Improving cancer patients hospital-home transition. Unpublished nursing research grant NR01493, National Center for Nursing Research, National Institutes of Health.

Padilla, G.F., & Grant, M.M. (1985). Quality of life as a cancer nursing outcome variable. *Advances in Nursing Science, 8*(1), 45–60.

Padilla, G.V., & Grant, M.M. (1987). Cancer nursing research, Chapter 44. In Groenwald, S.L. (Ed.), *Cancer nursing: Principles and practice,* Boston: Jones & Bartlett Publishers, Inc. 827–853.

Padilla, G.V., Presant, C.A., Grant, M.M., et al. (1983). Quality of life index for patients with cancer. *Research in Nursing and Health, 6,* 117–126.

Stetz, K.M., Lewis, F.M., Primomo, J. (1986). Family coping strategies and chronic illness in the mother. *Family Relations, 35,* 515–522.

CHAPTER 2

Progress In Cancer Nursing Research

Geraldine V. Padilla

During the first half of the 1980s there appeared a series of articles on the development and current status of cancer nursing research (Benoliel, 1983; Degner, 1984; Fernsler, Holcombe, & Pulliam, 1984; Grant & Padilla, 1983; Hilkemeyer, 1982; McCorkle & Lewis, 1980). Once a critical mass of cancer nursing studies had accumulated, scientists and editors felt it was time to review the progress that had been made, to evaluate the strengths and weaknesses of these investigations, and to provide direction for future endeavors. The present discussion summarizes the information in these review articles and provides an update on the status of cancer nursing research.

HISTORICAL DEVELOPMENT

Development of Nursing Research

The historical development of cancer nursing research closely parallels the emergence of scientific investigation in nursing and the expansion of medical research and specialization in cancer. The following summary of the emergence of nursing research is based on a report by Jeanne Quint Benoliel (1983).

After World War II, there began the serious movement of schools of nursing from hospitals to academic settings, changing the context of nurse training from apprenticeships to professional–scientific–clinical education. Academic values fostered the development of professional nursing, with research as an integral part of professionalization.

The decades of the 40s and 50s saw the birth of federal support for nursing research with the establishment of the Division of Nursing Resources in 1948 (later known as the Division of Nursing) and the appropriation of nursing research funds in 1955. These times also witnessed foundation support for nursing studies, as when Carnegie Foundation money led to the publication of *Nursing for the Future* by Esther Lucille Brown (1948). Other foundations that supported nursing education and service studies included the W.K. Kellogg and the Russell Sage Foundations. Doctoral education for nurses also began in earnest at this time: 132 nurses obtained doctoral degrees between 1926 and 1955. The Sigma Theta Tau Research fund began in 1934; the journal *Nursing Research* was first published in 1952 (Gortner & Nahm, 1977).

The sixties were characterized by continued development. For example, the American Nurses' Association undertook a major effort to support research. *Blueprint for Research in Nursing* and *The Nurse in Research — ANA Guidelines on Ethical Values* were first published in 1962 and 1968 respectively. The first ANA sponsored research conference took place in 1964; the first regional nursing research conference took place in 1968 under the sponsorship of the Western Interstate Commission on Education. The Sigma Theta Tau scholarly publication, *Image,* first appeared in 1967. Scientific training of nurses received major support in 1962 with the establishment of the Nurse Scientist Training Grants. These grants allowed nurses to participate in graduate programs that combined nursing with biomedical or behavioral disciplines. During this decade 449 doctorates were conferred on nurses, expanding the pool of qualified nurse scientists capable of conducting research and of training other nurse scientists.

By the 1970s and 80s, research was firmly established as a valued nursing activity. The ANA established the Commission on Nursing Research in 1970, and later the Council of Nurse Researchers. Twenty-two new doctoral programs for nurses were established throughout the United States. Three new journals dedicated to research were launched: *Research in Nursing and Health, Advances in Nursing Science,* and *Western Journal for Nursing Research.* Finally, in 1985, Congress established a National Center for Nursing Research within the National Institutes of Health (NIH). Dr Ada Sue Hinshaw is its first director.

Roots of Cancer Nursing Research

Hilkemeyer (1982) traced the medical, scientific, and technological advances in cancer knowledge and treatment. She noted that advances were fostered by federal and private support for cancer research. At present, federal support is concentrated in the National Cancer Institute (NCI), whereas private support comes largely from agencies such as the American Cancer Society.

The National Chemotherapy Section of NIH was established in 1956 and was followed by the formation of Cooperative Groups, whose purpose is promoting collaboration in the study of the impact of cancer chemotherapy as a treatment modality. The 1950s and 60s brought advances in chemotherapy, immunotherapy, hemotherapy, antibiotics, nutritional support, and bone marrow transplantation. Legislation in 1965 made grant monies available for the study of rehabilitation strategies for the cancer patient, infusing energy into that area of care. The National Cancer Act of 1971 and the revision of it in 1974 initiated a broad program to reduce the incidence, morbidity, and mortality of cancer. Major advances in cancer diagnosis, treatment, control, and delivery of health-care services can be traced to this important legislation, since it greatly increased basic research, led to the establishment of comprehensive cancer centers, supported complex medical protocols, and fostered nationwide study groups. As a consequence of these advances, many hospital oncology units and numerous community cancer rehabilitation and control programs have been established. In the 1970s and 80s the National Cancer Institute intensified its effort to promote the scientific basis of cancer care with the establishment of community-based programs such as the Clinical Hospital Oncology Programs (CHOPS) and the Community Clinical Oncology Programs (CCOPS). The 1980s witnessed growing support for multidisciplinary cancer research to decrease morbidity and mortality in high-risk, minority, and educationally and economically disadvantaged populations. Paralleling these federal efforts are those of private foundations such as the American Cancer Society.

Nurses have actively participated in medical research protocols. Initially, their role was confined to implementation of studies and data collection. Occasionally nurses provided input regarding procedural strategies to maintain the integrity of a study. These protocol nurses were seen as careful, cautious, and noninfluential participants in the research effort (McCorkle & Lewis, 1980). This was the usual manner in which cancer nurses were introduced to research. However, the passive role did not suit many nurses. It was inevitable that nursing committees within Cooperative Groups and Comprehensive Cancer Centers would seek greater active participation in the medical protocols.

The development of nurse-initiated cancer nursing research is traced through the following landmark studies reviewed by Hilkemeyer (1982). An early study conducted in 1947 reported that the cost of cancer nursing care was high. Results were used to establish financial support by the American Cancer Society, Connecticut Division (Biehusen, 1956). In 1953 Farrell reported on an experiment in teaching cancer nursing in four colleges (Farrell, 1953). In 1956 Gordon reviewed the nursing care records of new cancer cases in Nassau County, New York, to establish criteria for a cancer service (Gordon, 1956). Jeanne Quint later (1963) reported that a mastectomy tended to result in shock, change in physical appearance, and concern over a shortened life and a slow, painful death. Contrary to expectations, Quint's qualitative study showed that although surgical treatment for breast cancer was successful, patients found it very difficult to adjust to life changes caused by mastectomy. One of the first nursing studies on dying patients and pain control was carried out by Barckley (1964). An often-quoted study of cancer nursing research priorities was conducted by Oberst (1978). The study used the Delphi survey technique with 575 nurses and established that the highest research priorities related to problems of patients' physiological responses to treatment, i.e., chemotherapy, physical discomfort, and pain. The most important research priorities in nursing practice were identified as the need for organized support systems for the clinician, for education and for communication.

Hilkemeyer (1982) also outlined important events that have contributed to the development of cancer nursing research. The first time a nurse headed a Scientific Review Committee for the National Cancer Institute was between 1955 and 1957 when Hilkemeyer was appointed as chair of the Intervention Programs Review Committee. Beginning in the 1970s, nurses have had continuous representation on the Cancer Control Grant Review Committee of the NCI. Cancer nursing research grant applications have competed successfully in this arena. In 1975 the first Cancer Nursing Research Conference was sponsored by the American Cancer Society, California Division, together with the University of California, Los Angeles, School of Nursing and the University of California, San Francisco, Department of Continuing Education in Nursing.

The 1980s saw some important advances as well. For example, the Oncology Nursing Society established a research committee in 1980. The NCI inaugurated pre- and postdoctoral research training awards for nurses, with the first awards going to the University of Washington School of Nursing under the direction of Ruth McCorkle. The NCI also recognized the importance of research into cancer nursing problems when an oncology nurse, Anne Bavier, was appointed in 1986 to develop research in that area. The first nursing-focused Request for Applications (RFA) developed by Bavier was issued in 1986 and addressed nursing problems associated with home care of cancer patients. This handful of examples of the most recent developments in cancer nursing research is not meant to be all-inclusive but rather to represent the progress being made.

PRODUCTIVITY

Quantity and Focus of Published Research

The article by Fernsler, Holcombe, and Pulliam (1984) provides a helpful summary of the quantity and focus of cancer nursing research from January 1975 to June 1982. Only the nine journals that were expected to include cancer nursing research reports were reviewed. In 1975, five of these nine journals were in existence: *International Journal of Nursing Studies, Journal of Obstetric, Gynecologic, and Neonatal Nursing, Nursing Research, Oncology Nursing Forum*, and *Pediatric Nursing*. In 1976 *The American Journal of Maternal Child Nursing* was added. *Cancer Nursing* and *Research in Nursing and Health* first appeared in 1978. And *Western Journal of Nursing Research* began publication in 1979. Of the 1919 articles surveyed, 70 were considered cancer nursing studies because they had a nurse author or coauthor, focused on cancer nursing practice or education, included information about the research problem, hypothesis, or purpose, described a methodology, sample, and data analysis procedure, and stated findings. In a seven-and-a-half-year period, 9.6 percent of the articles published in these nine nursing journals were considered cancer nursing studies.

As expected, the bulk of cancer nursing investigations were published in *Cancer Nursing* (32), *Oncology Nursing Forum* (18) and *Nursing Research* (16). A few came from *Journal of Obstetric, Gynecologic, and Neonatal Nursing* (3), and *Western Journal of Nursing Research* (1). Between 1976 and 1978 the number of yearly cancer nursing research articles increased from one to ten with the addition of *Cancer Nursing* and *Research in Nursing and Health*. By 1981 yearly publications numbered 22 (Fernsler, Holcombe, & Pulliam, 1984).

The majority of studies focused on the client (50), some on the nurse (16), and a few on both (4). Of the studies that focused on the client, 31 investigated emotional and interpersonal behaviors, 19 studied biological responses, 8 addressed cancer prevention or detection, and 1 looked at the social aspects associated with cancer. Of the studies that investigated the nurse, 13 evaluated attitudes, 2 focused on knowledge, and 1 was concerned with both attitude and knowledge. None investigated nurse skills (Fernsler, Holcombe, & Pulliam, 1984). Information regarding the specific references belonging in each of the above categories may be obtained by contacting Dr Fernsler directly. At this writing, Dr Fernsler is associated with the University of Delaware College of Nursing.

A second article by Grant and Padilla (1983) provides similar information on quantity and focus for the period between 1970 and 1982. Sources used included: *International Nursing Index, Cumulative Index to Nursing and Allied Health Literature, Nursing Research, Communicating Nursing Research, Research in Nursing and Health, Western Journal of Nursing Research, Cancer Nursing, Oncology Nursing Forum,* and proceedings of major conferences on nursing and cancer nursing research. Also included were a few studies published in non-nursing journals as well as some in progress. Over 3000 studies were reviewed, with 328 categorized as cancer nursing studies. Selection was based on criteria similar to those used by Fernsler, Holcombe, and Pulliam. A list of these cancer nursing studies classified by topic can be obtained by writing to Dr Marcia Grant at the City of Hope National Medical Center in Duarte, California.

Studies in cancer nursing tended to focus on oncology nursing knowledge relevant to patient welfare (275) or on oncology nurses (53). According to Grant and Padilla, studies concerned with oncology nursing knowledge address the individual and family, health-illness continuum, health-care system, or community and environment. Within each of these categories studies were classified according to the "Outcome Standards for Cancer Nursing Education" published by the Oncology Nursing Society (1982).

The majority of oncology nursing knowledge studies reviewed dealt with the health-illness continuum (149). Common research problems in this category included care specific to individual cancer therapy, nausea and vomiting, nutrition, pain, patient teaching regarding therapy, and breast self-examination. Less common research topics were cancer detection, public education and prevention, diagnostic test preparation, oral problems, and complications. Neglected out-come standards included cancer risk and incidence factors, teaching the impor-tance of diagnostic and staging procedures, and unconventional treatment op-tions. The second major category of studies (92) focused on the individual and family. Here, the most common research questions dealt with psychosocial problems, family wellness, terminal care, quality of life, and stress associated with cancer patients. Less common topic areas included body image, breast reconstruction, rehabilitation, spiritual responses, financial, cultural, and hope-fulness factors. Fewer studies were found in the category of community and environment (19). However, the most popular research topics in this category were associated with home and hospice care. Poorly addressed outcome stan-dards in this category were those concerning carcinogens in the home, work, or community, and political factors. The health-care system category contained the fewest studies (15). Research questions in this last category addressed roles, compliance with therapy, students with cancer, and informed consent. Neglected outcome standards were components of the health-care system associated with cancer care, as well as legal, moral, and ethical issues related to cancer nursing care.

Studies concerned with oncology nurses (53) fell under five different head-ings: cancer unit characteristics and nursing care patterns (2), nurse attitudes toward cancer patients' death, cancer nursing care or cancer nurses (33), stress reduction for oncology nurses (6), quality assurance and standards of care in oncol-ogy nursing (4), and knowledge and education needs of oncology nurses (8).

Degner (1984) conducted a survey of 121 Canadian cancer centers, schools of nursing in university settings, and Victorian Order of Nurses agencies. Fifty-two questionnaires were returned. The best response rates were from schools of nursing and cancer centers. Of the 52 responding institutions, 32 stated that they were not currently conducting cancer nursing research. The 20 conducting such research identified 40 individual projects.

An analysis of the 40 research projects showed that 31 focused on patient welfare, 5 on nurse welfare, and 4 on other topics. These projects fell into the following research areas: psychological support of patients and families (9), discharge planning and follow-up programs (5), programs and policies affecting the dying (4), patient education material and methods (4), quality of life (3), stomatitis (2), relaxation therapy (2), staff attitudes (2), assisting patients to cope with grief (1), rights of dying patients (1), psychological impact on and support ·
for oncology staff (1), assisting nurses to cope with grief, loss, frustration (1), nursing education regarding specific treatment modalities and nursing tech-niques (1), and 4 others not categorized (Degner, 1984).

Quality of Published Research

Significance of the Research Question. The significance of research ques-tions addressed in cancer nursing studies can be measured against stated values of oncology nurses. These values appear as standards offered by the Oncology

Nursing Society and as research priorities identified by practicing oncology nurses. In the latter case, the review by Fernsler, Holcombe, and Pulliam (1984) found that of the 70 cancer nursing studies identified, only 19 addressed biological responses. The questions most commonly focused on were the emotional and interpersonal factors associated with cancer. This means that insufficient attention had been paid to the area of physiological responses to treatment, considered the highest research priority (Oberst, 1978).

Grant and Padilla (1983) found that of the 328 cancer nursing studies identified, 275 addressed a specific Oncology Nursing standard. The largest number of studies addressed standards related to the health–illness continuum. Of the 12 standards found in this area, 5 had not been studied by cancer nursing investigators and appeared more within the purview of epidemiologists, basic scientists, and physicians. Studies of the remaining seven standards addressed significant cancer nursing problems. Each of the standards related to the individual and family received the attention of one or more studies, with the largest cluster dealing with psychosocial responses and nursing interventions. The most underrepresented standards were those related to the health-care system, the community, and environment. Since these standards should also command the attention of investigators, Degner's recommendation for programmatic cancer nursing research (1984) seems very appropriate. A programmatic approach might ensure that certain oncology standards are not excluded from the research enterprise.

Significance is also measured by a study's contribution to knowledge. Of the 70 cancer nursing studies reviewed by Fernsler, Holcombe, and Pulliam, 23 reports included explicit information about the conceptual or theoretical framework for the study, whereas only 14 related findings back to the conceptual or theoretical framework. Ten reports stated explicit assumptions, 17 discussed limitations, and 33 reported on generalizability (Fernsler, Holcombe, & Pulliam, 1984). The lack of conceptualization together with the underreporting of assumptions, limitations, and generalizability suggests that scientific progress may be slow. The foundation of a scientific discipline is as strong as its theoretical structures. Without conceptual or theoretical frameworks to guide them, cancer nursing investigators may be lost in a sea of unrelated findings. McCorkle and Lewis (1980) recommend the development of frameworks that integrate concepts from a number of disciplines, while Hilkemeyer (1982) recommends collaborative research. Both approaches may contribute to stronger conceptualizations, which in turn contribute to the methodological rigor critical to knowledge growth (Grant & Padilla, 1983).

Scientific Rigor of the Methodology. Methodology is discussed in the review provided by Fernsler, Holcombe, and Pulliam (1984). Of the 70 cancer nursing articles found, 55 studies were descriptive, 14 were experimental or quasi-experimental, and 1 was historical. The authors conclude that the large number of descriptive studies indicates that cancer nursing research is in its early stages of development. Although the summary of cancer nursing studies provided by Grant and Padilla (1983) did not include a critique of methodology, the authors observed a need for more rigorous designs characterized by validity, generalizability, sensitivity, and efficiency. In those areas where little research has been found, well-designed exploratory studies are recommended; whereas problem areas already addressed by a few studies would benefit from randomized, prospective investigations that control relevant variables (Grant & Padilla, 1983).

With regard to data collection approaches, 47 used questionnaires, 5 used interviews, 5 used observations, and 13 used a combination of techniques. At least 55 studies used some form of investigator-devised instruments. Pilot testing of tools was mentioned in only 17 cases. Information on both reliability and validity was included in 15 reports, whereas data on either reliability or validity was presented in only 10 articles. This means that 45 reports did not include information on the reliability or validity of data-collection tools. Although the lack of information on reliability and validity of instruments is not conclusive proof of an actual deficiency, it does indicate a lack of appreciation for methodological rigor on the part of investigators and editors. These deficiencies speak poorly for the quality of the research. Though every new study should reevaluate the reliability and validity of its data-collection instruments, use of previously tested tools is an efficient way to increase the quality of a study.

Sample sizes ranged from under 10 to over 1000, with 60 percent of the studies having sample sizes of 50 or less. Whether small or large, the sample size should be justified. Power calculations or some other form of rationale for the size of the sample was missing from most reports. Most of the samples were composed of adult patients obtained from hospitals and clinics.

FUTURE DIRECTIONS IN CANCER NURSING RESEARCH

Recommendations for the 80s Based on Research in the 70s

A companion report to the Grant and Padilla (1983) article is the chapter by Padilla and Grant (1987) in the book, *Cancer Nursing: Principles and Practice.* Padilla and Grant (1987) provide some detail about the cancer nursing studies summarized in the earlier review of articles published in the 1970s or begun in the 1970s but published in the 1980s. Investigations are divided into five categories: (1) Population descriptors of cancer patients and nurses; (2) the impact of the cancer diagnosis; (3) the impact of cancer treatment, (4) the impact of the cancer prognosis; and (5) cancer and death education for patients and nurses. For each of these five categories of investigation, the authors recommend directions for future research based on needed areas of study neglected in the 1970s. Specific references for the types of studies identified below may be found in Padilla and Grant (1987).

Three methodological recommendations apply to all aspects of cancer nursing research. Future studies should be based on sound theoretical frameworks that are relevant to practice and integrated from a variety of related disciplines

(McCorkle & Lewis, 1980). In addition, increased methodological rigor is needed to produce research designs characterized by validity, generalizability, sensitivity, and efficiency (Padilla & Grant, 1987). Further, cancer nursing studies should be replicated before findings are applied to populations at large (Fernsler, Holcombe, and Pulliam, 1984). The need for replication before large scale use was emphasized by Horsley, Crane, and Bingle (1978).

Population Descriptors. In the category of population descriptors were found studies based on questionnaire surveys, interviews with patients, and reviews of medical records. These studies described various populations of cancer patients in terms of demographics, attitudes, cultural behaviors, stress, etc. Other studies described the oncology nurse in terms of education, role perception, job satisfaction, attitudes toward cancer and death, and stress and coping. It was recommended that future studies focus on current and projected needs for oncology nurses, the incidence of patient care problems specific to cancer, and epidemiologic studies related to cancer nursing (Padilla & Grant, 1987).

Impact of Cancer Diagnosis. Studies of the impact of the cancer diagnosis focusing on psychosocial aspects generally described the impact of a cancer diagnosis on patients and families. Specific attention was given to the impact of a diagnosis of breast cancer, lung cancer, or lymphoma. Studies of the physiological impact of a cancer diagnosis focused on such topic areas as diagnostic testing, pain, and enteral tube feeding. It was recommended that studies of blame and guilt about the diagnosis experienced by patients and families focus on the extent of the problem and strategies for alleviating it. Also needed were descriptions of the changing psychosocial impact of the cancer diagnosis and healthy coping mechanisms that would be relevant to the changing problems. Additional studies were needed on nursing interventions to alleviate pain, teaching to promote patient and family pain care management, and effectiveness of pain control through analgesia, relaxation, and biofeedback. Also important were nutrition studies of nursing approaches to alleviate cachexia, anorexia, and taste changes as well as studies of the impact of cancer on physical activities, energy expenditure related to specific physical activities, and strategies for achieving maximum activity levels while not aggravating weight loss (Padilla & Grant, 1987).

Impact of Cancer Treatment. In this category, a relatively larger number of studies on the psychosocial impact of treatment was found, indicating the importance of this area of research in oncology nursing. These studies dealt with the general effects of hospitalization and cancer treatment, the specific effects of treatment approaches such as germ-free environments or mastectomy, the effects of nursing care approaches such as comfort measures, and compliance of patients in different treatment regimens. Publications related to the physiological impact of cancer treatment revealed a growing interest in the effect of various medical treatment modalities on patient care problems. Some problems, such as mouth care, were well developed and included valid tools, and laboratory and clinical evidence. Several studies focused on cancer nursing and quality of care. It was recommended that future research continue to address the problems associated with hospitalization, isolation, disfiguring surgery, debilitating medical treatment, the stress associated with treatment, and ways of alleviating the stress. Since there is a paucity of information regarding disruptions in sleep and sexual activity, attention to these problems was recommended. Studies of personal and environmental selective neglect of cancer patients by staff are very important because such behavior may be viewed by families as examples of nursing's lack of compassion or as loss of control or independence. With regard to the physiological impact of treatment, studies are needed on preoperative care of different surgical populations, ongoing care of patients with different devices such as ostomy apparatus, and continuing care of patients suffering side effects of therapy. Studies are also needed to identify standards of oncology nursing care, to develop tools to measure and implement these standards, and to measure the impact of these standards on patient welfare (Padilla & Grant, 1987).

Impact of Cancer Prognosis. The area of the psychosocial impact of the cancer prognosis included studies on nurses' attitudes and beliefs about death and dying, their behavior toward patients with terminal prognoses, and the support needs of families, patients, and nurses. The investigation of the impact of the cancer prognosis on health-care delivery systems has included studies on hospice care, radiation oncology outpatient nursing care, community oncology clinical specialists, needs of patients and families in the home environment, and the relative costs of home and hospital care. Future research is needed to accurately assess the needs of dying patients, the nursing care required for terminal patients in the hospital and home, and the nursing care for patients in different age groups and from diverse cultural backgrounds. The postdeath care needed by families of cancer patients should be investigated along with the role of oncology nurses in facilitating decisions for the terminally ill. The effect of experience with terminal care on the nurse's development of sympathy toward, comfortableness with, and callousness regarding dying patients should also be studied. Little information regarding the physiological impact of a cancer prognosis has been found in nursing research. Thus, this area of investigation requires immediate attention. Kinds of studies needed include descriptions of the incidence of physical problems characteristic of terminal care, and the impact of these problems on the length and quality of life. Some common problems are skin care, pain, disorientation, fractures, infections, bleeding, thirst, wound odor, lymphedema, and communication, to name a few. The area of impact of cancer prognosis also needs research on systems of care delivery. Additional studies are needed on home versus hospice care, on costs of these nursing services, and on interventions that are economical yet address the physical and psychological needs of the patients (Padilla & Grant, 1987).

Cancer and Death Education. Cancer and death education studies focused on the consumer or patient as well as the nurse. Consumer and patient education studies included research that sought to influence health practices and experimental and nonexperimental descriptions and evaluations of knowledge and skill learning programs, including breast cancer detection and support groups. Nurse education studies focused on roles and expectations of cancer education teachers, on the learning needs of oncology nurses, on the cancer and death education programs available to nurses, and the coping and support needs of oncology nurses. Research needs to continue with education programs to improve nursing knowledge, assessment, and intervention skills regarding specific types of cancer other than breast tumors, available treatments, and types of information and personality variables that promote compliance with cancer treatment while reducing the distress associated with treatment and side effects. Cost-effective factors related to education should be measured because education may impact on prevention, hospitalization, self-care, and adaptation to diagnosis and treatment. Finally, it is recommended that studies examining the relationship of actual, recorded patient teaching behaviors to patient learning outcomes be conducted (Padilla & Grant, 1987).

Several areas of cancer nursing research appear to be outside the five categories of studies described above yet deserve special mention because of their growing interest and importance. These include basic research efforts related to cancer nursing, spiritual aspects of cancer care, the role of nurses in clinical trials, the implementation of cancer nursing research through cooperative groups, and problems in applying nursing research findings to oncology practice (Padilla & Grant, 1987).

Cancer Nursing Research Midway through the 80s

An analysis of the 1986 issues of *Cancer Nursing, Oncology Nursing Forum, Nursing Research, Research in Nursing and Health, Western Journal of Nursing Research,* and *Advances in Nursing Science* yielded the following information about research focuses during that year. The three research journals published 120 scientific articles, excluding features, editorials, and the like. Of these 120 articles, 8 (6.6 percent) were considered to be cancer nursing research since they dealt with oncology patients, oncology nursing problems, or hospice care. The two cancer journals published 79 articles, excluding features, editorials, etc. Of these 79, 40 (50.6 percent) were identified as scientific investigations.

The 48 cancer nursing research articles published in the five journals listed above included 4 tool development studies; 3 descriptive program evaluation studies; 27 one-group descriptive studies and 9 two- or three-group comparison descriptive studies, very few of which made use of a random selection procedure, and 5 experimental or quasi-experimental studies. Data collection covered periods of six months or less. Units of analysis were patients (27 studies), families or caregivers (4 studies), nurses (15 studies), healthy subjects (5), and agencies (2). Some studies included more than one type of unit of analysis. Numbers of subjects ranged from 1 agency (Clark, 1986) whose day hospital for cancer patients was being evaluated to 823 nurses (Feldman & Richard, 1986) who returned a mailed survey on prevalence and quit rate of smoking-related behaviors. Diagnoses of patients participating in these research studies were not always stated. Mail-out–mail-return surveys were conducted as part of five studies. The return rates for these surveys were quite good ranging from 46 percent (Dalton & Swenson, 1986) to 88 percent (Gritz & Kanim, 1986) with the mean at 63 percent.

Population Descriptors. Using the same classification system as found in Padilla and Grant (1987), the first group of five studies is concerned with descriptions of populations of clients: social network and support perceived by Swiss cancer patients (Kesselring, Lindsey, Dodd, & Lovejoy, 1986); health beliefs about testicular cancer self-examination among professional men (Blesch, 1986); perceived susceptibility to breast cancer and practice of breast self-examination (Massey, 1986); knowledge of cancer among elderly individuals (Weinrich & Weinrich, 1986); and knowledge of diagnosis, management program, and risks of therapy among new patients with ovarian cancer (Karani & Wiltshaw, 1986). A second group of eight population descriptor studies focuses on the nurse: influence of cultural background of African versus Midwestern-American nurses on attitudes and care of oncology patients (Martin & Belcher, 1986) cancer nurses' perceptions of caring (Larson, 1986); personal and professional aspects of the nurse–patient relationship (Trygstad, 1986); burnout in oncology nurses (Jenkins & Ostchega, 1986); nurses' attitudes toward sexuality in cancer patients (Williams, et al, 1986); and nurses and smoking (Feldman & Richard, 1986; Gritz & Kanim, 1986; Dalton & Swenson, 1986).

Impact of Cancer Diagnosis. Two areas are covered under this heading. The first topic area includes six studies on the psychosocial impact of cancer: nurse perceptions of the impact of the diagnosis on prognosis for oncology and coronary heart disease patients (Solodky, et al, 1986); needs of cancer patients (Derdiarian, 1986) and their families (Tringali, 1986); impact of a cancer diagnosis on Swiss patients and their families (Kesselring, Dodd, Lindsey, & Strauss, 1986); on sexual adjustment (Waterhouse & Metcalfe, 1986); and on managing one's life with melanoma (Longman & Graham, 1986). The second topic area covers the physiological impact of cancer: on perceptions of dyspnea in lung cancer patients (Brown, et al, 1986); critical variables associated with the pain experience (Bressler, Hange, & McGuire, 1986; Austin, et al, 1986); non-analgesic methods of pain control (Barbour, McGuire, & Kirchhoff, 1986); and continuous subcutaneous infusion (Coyle, et al, 1986).

Impact of Cancer Treatment. Psychosocial impact includes investigations of family responses to hospitalization (Lovejoy, 1986); patient and nurse perceptions of self-care deficits associated with chemotherapy (Fernsler, 1986); coping and adaptation in women receiving chemotherapy for breast cancer (Hopkins, 1986); late effects of central nervous system prophylactic treatment for leukemia on cognitive functioning (Moore, Kramer, & Ablin, 1986); effects of glucocorticosteroid treatment on depression and life style (Post-White, 1986); the influence of anxiety (Rhodes, Watson, & Johnson, 1986) or of relaxation versus an antiemetic drug regimen (Scott, et al, 1986) on nausea and vomiting during chemotherapy. The physiological impact of treatment includes studies on protective measures for nurses handling parenteral antineoplastic agents (Stajich, et al, 1986); symptom distress in patients receiving Texol (Strauman, 1986); taste changes in patients undergoing radiotherapy or combination chemotherapy (Huldij, et al, 1986); and moisture vapor dressings compared to conventional dressings for management of radiation skin reactions (Shell, Stanutz, & Grimm, 1986). Some investigations have also focused on standards of care in relation to measures of patient satisfaction (LaMonica, et al, 1986); to the relationship between task complexity, nursing expertise, and the planning process for pain management (Corcoran, 1986); and to nursing practices regarding the teaching of breast self-examination (Sawyer, 1986).

Impact of Cancer Prognosis. Studies in this area examined the psychosocial impact of prognosis as well as health-care delivery systems. In the case of the former, Holing (1986) described the primary caregiver's perception of the dying trajectory; Francis (1986) explored the concerns of Hindu cancer patients; and Reed (1986) examined differences in religiousness among terminally ill adults. Health-care delivery was analyzed in relation to the clinical and economical feasibility of a day hospital for cancer patients (Clark, 1986) and hospice and home care for dying children (Hays, 1986; Lauer, et al, 1986; Martinson, et al, 1986).

Cancer and Death Education. One study investigated the effect of an education program on the knowledge and attitudes of nurses regarding cancer pain management (Hauck, 1986). A second study evaluated a program that addressed the informational and emotional concerns of cancer patients and their families (Fredette & Beattie, 1986). A third study compared the impact of group versus individual teaching of breast self-examination to working women on their knowledge, beliefs, and self-examination practices (Brailey, 1986).

SUMMARY

This section on future directions in cancer nursing research has illustrated the value of categorizing articles to determine whether past recommendations are reflected in present research trends. A comparison of the author's review of 1986 publications with recommendations for future research published in Padilla and Grant (1987) indicates where studies are still needed. The reader should bear in mind that all recommendations reflect a personal viewpoint and are necessarily limited by the biases of the author.

1. Descriptive studies of patient care questions continue to form the bulk of cancer nursing research efforts and are likely to continue throughout the 1980s.

2. Recommended population descriptor studies on nurse needs and incidence of patient care problems were published in 1986.
3. Recommended studies on the impact of the cancer diagnosis in relation to pain control and adjustment are found in 1986 publications. However, studies on blame and guilt are still needed as are studies on nutrition, weight loss, and physical activity.
4. Recommended investigations related to the impact of treatment have included hospitalization, and cognitive, physical, and emotional side effects of therapy and standards of care. Lacking are studies on disruptions in sleep and sexual activity and neglect of cancer patients.
5. Recommended studies on the impact of cancer prognosis in relation to needs of dying patients and alternative care systems for these patients were published in 1986. There continues to be a paucity of information on physiological aspects of the dying process, related care, and quality of life.
6. Only three studies related to cancer and death education were identified in the author's review of 1986 cancer nursing research publications. There continues to be a need for investigating the cost of oncology nurse and patient education programs in relation to cancer prevention, hospitalization, self-care, and adaptation to illness. Also needed are studies that investigate the impact of patient and nurse education programs on desired patient and nurse behavioral outcomes.

REFERENCES

American Nurses' Association. (1962). ANA blueprint for research in nursing. *American Journal of Nursing, 62,* 69–71.

American Nurses' Association. (1968). *The nurse in research: ANA guidelines on ethical values.* New York: American Nurses' Association.

Austin, C., Eyres, P.J., Hefferin, E.A., et al (1986). Hospice home care pain management: Four critical variables. *Cancer Nursing, 9*(2), 58–65.

Barbour, L.A., McGuire, D.B., Kirchhoff, K.T. (1986). Nonanalgesic methods of pain control used by cancer outpatients. *Oncology Nursing Forum, 13*(6), 56–60.

Barckley, V. (1964). Enough time for good nursing. *Nursing Outlook, 12*(4), 44–48.

Benoliel, J.Q. (1983). The historical development of cancer nursing research in the United States. *Cancer Nursing, 5,* 261–267.

Biehusen, I. (1956). Cancer nursing is expensive. *Nursing Outlook, 4,* 438–441.

Blesch, J.S. (1986). Health beliefs about testicular cancer self-examination among professional men. *Oncology Nursing Forum, 13*(1), 29–33.

Brailey, L.J. (1986). Effects of health teaching in the workplace on women's knowledge, beliefs, and practices regarding breast self-examination. *Research in Nursing and Health, 9,* 223–231.

Bressler, L.R., Hange, P.A., McGuire, D.B. (1986). Characterization of the pain experience in a sample of cancer outpatients. *Oncology Nursing Forum, 13*(6), 51–55.

Brown, E.L. (1948). *Nursing for the future.* New York: Russell Sage Foundation.

Brown, M.L., Carrier, V., Janson-Bjerklie, S., et al (1986). Lung cancer and dyspnea: The patient's perception. *Oncology Nursing Forum, 13*(5), 19–24.

Clark, M. (1986). A day hospital for cancer patients: Clinical and economic feasibility. *Oncology Nursing Forum, 13*(6), 41–45.

Corcoran, S.A. (1986). Planning by expert and novice nurses in cases of varying complexity. *Research in Nursing and Health, 9,* 155–162.

Coyle, N., Mauskop, A., Maggard, J., et al (1986). Continuous subcutaneous infusions of opiates in cancer patients with pain. *Oncology Nursing Forum, 13*(4), 53–57.

Dalton, J.A., & Swenson, I. (1986). Nurses and smoking: Role modeling and counseling behaviors. *Oncology Nursing Forum, 13*(2), 45–48.

Degner, L.F. (1984). The status of cancer nursing research in Canada. *Nursing Papers, 16*(4), 4–13.

Derdiarian, A.K. (1986). Informational needs of recently diagnosed cancer patients. *Nursing Research, 35*(5), 276–281.

Farrell, M. (1953). Experimentation in teaching cancer nursing. *Nursing Research, 2*(1), 41.

Feldman, B.M., & Richard, E. (1986). Prevalence of nurse smokers and variables identified with successful and unsuccessful smoking cessation. *Research in Nursing and Health, 9,* 131–138.

Fernsler, J. (1986). A comparison of patient and nurse perceptions of patients' self-care deficits associated with cancer chemotherapy. *Cancer Nursing, 9*(2), 50–57.

Fernsler, J., Holcombe, J., Pulliam, L. (1984). A survey of cancer nursing research. *Oncology Nursing Forum, 11*(4), 46–52.

Francis, M. R. (1986). Concerns of terminally ill adult Hindu cancer patients. *Cancer Nursing, 9*(4), 164–171.

Fredette, S.L., & Beattie, H.M. (1986). Living with cancer: A patient education program. *Cancer Nursing, 9*(6), 308–316.

Gordon, D.E. (1956). Appraising a cancer service: A study to establish criteria. *Public Health Reports, 71,* 399–407.

Gortner, S.R., & Nahm, H. (1977). An overview of nursing research in the United States. *Nursing Research, 26,* 10–33.

Grant, M.M., & Padilla, G.V. (1983). An overview of cancer nursing research. *Oncology Nursing Forum, 10*(1), 58–67.

Gritz, E.R., & Kanim, L. (1986). Do fewer oncology nurses smoke? *Oncology Nursing Forum, 13*(3), 61–64.

Hauck, S.L. (1986). Pain: Problem for the person with cancer. *Cancer Nursing, 9*(2), 66–76.

Hays, J.C. (1986). Patient symptoms and family coping: Predictors of hospice utilization patterns. *Cancer Nursing, 9*(6), 317–325.

Hilkemeyer, R. (1982). Update on nursing issues: A historical perspective on cancer nursing. *Oncology Nursing Forum, 9*(2), 47–56.

Holing, E.V. (1986). The primary caregiver's perception of the dying trajectory: An exploratory study. *Cancer Nursing, 9*(1), 29–37.

Hopkins, M.B. (1986). Information-seeking and adaptational outcomes in women receiving chemotherapy for breast cancer. *Cancer Nursing, 9*(1), 256–262.

Horsley, J.A., Crane, J., Bingle, J.D. (1978). Research utilization as an organizational process. *Journal of Nursing Administration, 8,* 4–6.

Huldij, A., Giesbers, A., Poelhuis, E.H.K., et al (1986). *Cancer Nursing, 9*(1), 38–42.

Jenkins, J.F., & Ostchega, Y. (1986). Evaluation of burnout in oncology nurses. *Cancer Nursing, 9*(3), 108–116.

Karani, D., & Wiltshaw, E. (1986). How well informed? *Cancer Nursing, 9*(5), 238–242.

Kesselring, A., Dodd, M.J., Lindsey, A.M., et al (1986). Attitudes of patients living in Switzerland about cancer and its treatment. *Cancer Nursing, 9*(2), 77–85.

Kesselring, A., Lindsey, A.M., Dodd, M.J., et al (1986). Social network and support perceived by Swiss cancer patients. *Cancer Nursing, 9*(4), 156–163.

LaMonica, E.L., Oberst, M.T., Madea, A.R., et al (1986). Development of a patient satisfaction scale. *Research in Nursing and Health, 9,* 43–50.

Larson, P.J. (1986). Cancer nurses' perceptions of caring. *Cancer Nursing, 9*(2), 86–91.

Lauer, M.E., Mulhern, R.K., Hoffman, R.G., et al (1986). Utilization of hospice/home care in pediatric oncology. *Cancer Nursing, 9*(3), 102–107.

Longman, A.J., & Graham, K.Y. (1986). Living with melanoma: Content analysis of interviews. *Oncology Nursing Forum, 13*(4), 58–64.

Lovejoy, N.C. (1986). Family responses to cancer hospitalization. *Oncology Nursing Forum, 13*(2), 33–37.

Martin, B.A., & Belcher, J.V. (1986). Influence of cultural background on nurses' attitudes and care of the oncology patient. *Cancer Nursing, 9*(5), 230–237.

Martinson, I.M., Moldow, D.G., Armstrong, G.D., et al (1986). Home care for children dying of cancer. *Research in Nursing and Health, 9,* 11–16.

Massey, V. (1986). Perceived susceptibility to breast cancer and practice of breast self-examination. *Nursing Research, 35*(3), 183–185.

McCorkle, R., & Lewis, F.M. (1980). Research in cancer nursing. *Seminars in Oncology, 7*(1), 80–87.

Moore, I.M., Kramer, J., Ablin, A. (1986). Late effects of central nervous system prophylactic leukemia therapy on cognitive functioning. *Oncology Nursing Forum, 13*(4), 45–51.

Oberst, M. (1978). Priorities in cancer nursing research. *Cancer Nursing, 1*(8), 281–290.

Oncology Nursing Society Education Committee. (1982). *Outcome standards for cancer nursing education.* Pittsburgh: Oncology Nursing Society.

Padilla, G.V., & Grant, M.M. (1987). Cancer nursing research. In S.L. Groenwald (Ed.), *Cancer nursing: Principles and practice* (827–853). Boston: Jones and Bartlett.

Post-White, J. (1986). Glucocorticosteroid-induced depression in the patient with leukemia or lymphoma. *Cancer Nursing, 9*(1), 15–22.

Quint, J.C. (1963). Impact of mastectomy. *American Journal of Nursing, 63*(11), 88–92.

Reed, P.G. (1986). Religiousness among terminally ill and healthy adults. *Research in Nursing and Health, 9,* 35–41.

Rhodes, V.A., Watson, P.M., Johnson, M.H. (1986). Association of chemotherapy related nausea and vomiting with pretreatment and posttreatment anxiety. *Oncology Nursing Forum, 13*(1), 41–47.

Sawyer, P.F. (1986). Breast self-examination: Hospital-based nurses aren't assessing their clients. *Oncology Nursing Forum, 13*(5), 44–48.

Scott, D.W. Donahue, D.C., Mastrovito, R.C., et al (1986). Comparative trial of clinical relaxation and an antiemetic drug regimen in reducing chemotherapy-related nausea and vomiting. *Cancer Nursing, 9*(4), 178–187.

Shell, J.A., Stanutz, F., Grimm, J. (1986). Comparison of moisture vapor permeable (MVP) dressings to conventional dressings for management of radiation skin reactions. *Oncology Nursing Forum, 13*(1), 11–16.

Solodky, M., Mikos, K., Bordieri, J., et al (1986). Nurses' prognosis for oncology and coronary heart disease patients. *Cancer Nursing, 9*(5), 243–247.

Stajich, G.V., Barnett, C.W., Turner, S.V., et al (1986). Protective measures used by oncologic office nurses handling parenteral antineoplastic agents. *Oncology Nursing Forum, 13*(6), 47–49.

Strauman, J.J. (1986). Symptom distress in patients receiving phase I chemotherapy with Taxol. *Oncology Nursing Forum, 13*(5), 40–43.

Tringali, C.A. (1986). The needs of family members of cancer patients. *Oncology Nursing Forum, 13*(4), 65–70.

Trygstad, L. (1986). Professional friends: The inclusion of the personal into the professional. *Cancer Nursing, 9*(6), 326–332.

Waterhouse, J., & Metcalfe, M.C. (1986). Development of the sexual adjustment questionnaire. *Oncology Nursing Forum, 13*(3), 53–59.

Weinrich, S.P., & Weinrich, M.C. (1986). Cancer knowledge among elderly individuals. *Cancer Nursing, 9*(6), 301–307.

Williams, H.A., Wilson, M.E., Hongladarom, G., et al (1986). Nurses' attitudes toward sexuality in cancer patients. *Oncology Nursing Forum, 13*(2), 39–43.

CHAPTER 3

Development of the Research Question

Ruth McCorkle

Few researchers would deny that the most critical step in the research process is the conceptual phase, which begins with the formulation of the research question. The research question is a series of statements containing interrelated elements of the problem, related concepts, and the purpose, which reflects the opinions and ideas of the researchers. The types of problems selected for study will vary from researcher to researcher. The purpose of this chapter is to present a framework to assist nurses in formulating research questions in cancer nursing, from the selection of the problem to the formulation of specific questions or hypotheses.

Clinical nursing offers researchers an opportunity to study diverse problems in a natural setting. Nurses who work with the day-to-day situations in which patients confront what is happening to them question a range of alternatives that may be useful in understanding, enhancing, or facilitating their experiences. It is common for nurses to question what happens to patients, why, and what can be done. The purpose of research is to answer questions that arise from curiosity or practical need (Schantz & Lindeman, 1982). Not all questions need to be studied systematically, but for those that do, nurses play a key role in formulating questions for research. "A research question is an explicit query about a problem or issue that can be challenged, examined, and analyzed, and that will yield useful new information" (Brink & Wood, 1983).

IDENTIFICATION OF NURSING PROBLEMS

Many nurses may think they are inept at identifying research problems or participating in the research process. In fact, they are active participants in evaluating the effectiveness of nursing care. Nurses have been taught to solve clinical problems by using the nursing process. The nursing process is a useful starting point for understanding the research process. Both processes are concerned with three basic questions: What is the problem? What are the response options? Do any or all of the response options solve the problem. The nursing process differs from research in that it focuses on the problems of one situation or patient at a time, whereas the research process is concerned with answering questions that are generalizable to a group of patients or events (Padilla, 1979). The nurses' background in solving clinical problems by using the nursing process is an excellent basis for formulating research questions.

According to Batey (1971), the research process has three phases; conceptual, empirical, and interpretative. The conceptual phase deals with the identification of research problems, the conceptual framework, prior knowledge about those problems, and the purpose. The empirical phase deals with the conduct of the study to obtain the information and to make sense of the facts to fulfill the purpose. The interpretative phase is the discovery of the meaning of the facts obtained in relation to the purpose and conceptual framework.

Focusing on Areas of Interest

There is an abundance of clinical nursing problems and there are several ways to facilitate the formation of a research problem. One of the most effective ways of identifying a significant question is through direct observations, thoughts, and experiences. A second method is by discussion with experienced nurses.

Many nurses have invented ways to help patients and to simplify routines. Both of these methods of identifying a research problem are illustrated in the following example.

> While attending graduate school, my first research problem evolved from working with a man experiencing a heart attack. I worked the night shift in an intensive care unit in a small community hospital. Often the unit was unoccupied, and one of the two nurses assigned to the unit would be transferred to assist elsewhere in the hospital. The on-call physician did not routinely stay in the hospital at night but was available as needed. One night, about halfway into the shift, a man was brought in by ambulance. The man, in his late 60s, was gasping for breath and clutching his chest with his hands. The man whispered he was in severe pain and pleaded for me to do something. His color was pale and he was extremely diaphoretic. The ambulance driver transferred the patient from the stretcher to the bed while I spoke to the physician to report the patient's status and obtain an order for a narcotic. The physician stated he was on his way and it would take about twenty minutes. He preferred not to

medicate him until he saw him. In the meantime, I was to proceed with the routine cardiac nursing procedures. The head of the bed was elevated and oxygen started; the man was connected to a cardiac monitor; an intravenous line was established and blood samples drawn. I had quickly and quietly completed these tasks and realized that the man had not improved. It seemed like an eternity since I had called the physician, but in fact it had only been several minutes. I was confronted with the feeling of "What do I do now?," alone with this man who was obviously dying before my eyes. I decided I could not just stand there. I pulled up a chair and sat with the man, holding his hand. I spoke to him by name, telling him I didn't know what was going to happen, but that I was with him and I wasn't going to leave. As I sat there, I stroked his hand and asked him to breathe with me. I sat quietly, stroking his hand, and looking at him. Within a few minutes, his breathing was less labored, his color improved, his diaphoresis lessened, and he seemed to be less anxious. When the physician arrived, he confirmed that the man had sustained a myocardial infarction and ordered medications to relieve his chest pain and to control his arrhythmia. The man survived and over the next several nights we spoke to each other about the experience and how powerful it had been. The man repeatedly told me I had saved his life.

The experience was a turning point in my career, and I wanted to use it as a basis for my research project. I began to openly discuss my nursing care with my peers. I wanted to know if other nurses had had similar experiences and what approaches they had used to comfort a patient who was obviously in crisis. I quickly validated that, in general, nurses thought their presence was comforting to patients, especially if touch was used. These discussions led me to formulate a research question for my graduate studies about the effects of touch on seriously ill patients. (McCorkle, 1974)

Another method of formulating a question is by reading the literature and recognizing discrepancies and gaps. For example, there may be a discrepancy between what is presented in an article and what actually occurs in the nurse's practice. The nurse may find her- or himself disagreeing with the author or thinking the author did not prove the point to the satisfaction of the reader. At this point a nurse may feel frustrated over the perceived discrepancy and wish to document the author's error. These discrepancies are an excellent basis for formulating a research question. For example, Saunders (1981) noted that the death of a loved one had been universally identified as unequalled in its capacity to cause personal pain and suffering. Previous research had demonstrated that survivors experience a wide range of feeling and behaviors, including numbness, depression, restlessness, and crying. A great deal was known about the somatic responses of widows, but little was known about the widow's social relationships with others. Saunders' experience led her to believe, however, that there in fact might be some circumstances in which death is seen as a relief. She studied a number of unanswered questions about the survivors' interpersonal responses to the death of a spouse: Did widows' responses differ according to the mode of death (natural, accidental, suicidal, or homicidal)? Did mode of death influence changes in widows social interactions as well as their physical and psychological responses?

A fourth way of identifying a research problem is by evaluating the logic of and scientific support for a theory about a particular substantive field. Lewis' work on personal control (1982) illustrates how a research question can be generated from a published theory.

The idea of control has been conceptualized within a reinforcement paradigm by both Rotter's social learning theory (1964) and Seligman's theory of helplessness (1975). From these theories, Lewis hypothesized that perceived self worth is related to a sense of control over the current life situation. Lewis stated that little is known about the meaning of experienced personal control as it relates to quality of life in late-stage cancer patients. She predicted that maximizing the cancer patient's sense of personal control results in the experience of a better quality of life.

In summary, four methods that a nurse can use to identify a research problem include: (1) direct observations, thoughts, and experience; (2) discussion with experienced nurses; (3) reading the literature and recognizing discrepancies; and (4) evaluating a theory about a substantive field. Once a nursing problem has been identified, the next step is to develop the research questions from an analysis of the problem.

Characteristics of a Problem

Usually the problem statement is a single sentence that describes the variables of interest in broad terms, possibly the relationship among those variables, and the population in which the variables are being studied. This statement can be in declarative or interrogative form and, when well-written, will suggest the specific hypothesis or research question that the study will address. It should also suggest the appropriate research design that is needed to answer the question(s) asked.

In its completed form, the phenomenon to be addressed by a study is referred to varyingly in the research literature as the objective, the research problem, or the research purpose. Regardless of the label used to denote it, this is what sets the context of the study. It is the unit of presentation that seems to introduce the study by setting its major parameters (Batey, 1977).

Lindeman and Schantz (1982) recommend that the researcher begin by writing an unedited statement of the problem. They emphasize *unedited* because a frequent stumbling block is the struggle to create a grammatically correct statement while holding on to a creative idea.

The revisions that are needed to change the nursing question into a researchable question are often extensive. The concepts need to be identified and defined. The factors that influence the problem need to be isolated. Benner (1984) suggests that the *aspects* of a situation are one form of clinical knowledge accessible only to the experienced nurse. One method of transforming the clinical problem into a research problem is to list the aspects of the situation and identify all the possible questions that need to be answered about the problem.

Wilson (1985) recommends that a four-step approach be used to arrive at research problems. In step one, the nurse clearly states the discrepancies that are observed in clinical practice. Next, the nurse needs to brainstorm all the plausible explanations or obstacles to describe the problem and its solution. Third, the nurse narrows the focus of the problem by limiting it to a few concepts that are critical. And fourth, the nurse rephrases the problem in words that reflect concepts that are measurable.

Justification and Significance of Problem

The next task is to decide what questions are the most important and feasible to answer. Clinical knowledge is used by the nurse in determining what problems need to be studied and which problems should have priority. Benner and Wrubel (1982) define clinical knowledge as that knowledge embedded in the practice of nursing. Clinical knowledge is critical to nursing practice to the extent that it makes a difference in patient outcomes.

The development of clinical knowledge is based on experience founded in systematic study and in clinical practice. Experience is not the mere passage of time, but "rather it is the transformation of preconceived notions and expectations by means of encounters with actual practical situations. Experience implies further that there is a dialogue between what is found in practice, or in the practical situation, and what is expected." (Benner & Wrubel, 1982, p. 11).

For a problem to become a researchable question, it must meet recognized criteria. Valiga and Mermel (1985) have identified several standards that they think must be met before the nurse proceeds in developing the study. First and most importantly, the question must be researchable. It must lead to "answers" through some form of data collection. A researchable question must be of interest to the investigator. Research is a time-consuming activity on the part of the research team, the subjects, and health-care systems. For the nurse to engage in research in which there is little or no interest jeopardizes the quality of the work and may bias the finding of the study.

Researchable questions should be feasible and practical to study. The nurse must consider the time involved to do the study, the cost, space, competence of the researcher, special resources, environment, support services, and the availability of subjects. The researcher must address the following questions: "Why study this problem?", "What difference will it make?", "Is it possible to study this problem?", and "What are the obstacles to implementing the study?" For example, the researcher may have developed an excellent research problem to study the effects on patients of receiving chemotherapy but be unable to implement the study because he or she lacks access to patients on chemotherapy. The researcher must also judge whether the study is feasible to do.

Feasibility refers to whether the study can be planned, implemented, and completed. Conditions that may interfere with the success of a study are: lack of time, money and space; inexperience of the investigator; need for special resources such as a one-way mirror to observe behavior; inaccessibility to essential data such as the medical record; unfriendly or hostile environment; and inadequate financial and/or administrative support (Fleming, 1984). In addition, the answers gained from research questions ultimately should have significance for nursing practice. The findings should add new knowledge to nursing science and ultimately improve the quality of nursing care. Significant research questions yield contributions to the science or the discipline of nursing in a meaningful way.

SELECTION OF A RESEARCHABLE NURSING PROBLEM

The problem statement is a summary statement of the phenomena to be investigated in relation to the answers needed (Lindsey, 1983). The content of the statement identifies the scope of the problem area, who's affected by the problem, and for how long. The words or concepts in the statement give direction to the literature to be searched for further clarification and specification of the problem. Literature citations for discrepancies between major aspects of the study are needed. The problem statement should also describe how nursing is affected by the phenomena and justify the importance of the phenomena.

A series of questions shown in Table 3–1 have been formulated to guide the nurse in identifying a research problem. It is recommended that the nurse answer the questions on the guide as an initial step in stating the problem.

After the researcher has identified one or two important questions, the context or domain of the problem should be made explicit. For example, in Padilla, Baker, and Dolan's study (1977) on interacting with dying patients, the domain of the study is the practice of caring for dying patients and their families. The study was generated by observing that nurses who care for the dying often feel inadequately prepared. The authors noted that nurses' attitudes toward death and dying are shaped by behaviors they learn during their formal education and early work experience. The study was designed to determine whether an educational program aimed at exploring prevailing attitudes and behaviors toward dying patients would help nurses become more comfortable and skillful in interacting with dying patients and, therefore, benefit patients. Nurses who cared for dying patients were reported as being anxious and avoiding patient contact. The researchers assumed nurses' anxiety was due to their inadequate formal preparation and poor role models. The subjects in their study were professional nurses. A more relevant index for nursing is the Cumulative Index to Nursing and Allied Health Literature.

REVIEW OF LITERATURE

After the researcher has an initial statement of the problem written, he or she proceeds to the literature. The concepts or words in the statement of the problem become the headings for searches through the published cumulative indices.

TABLE 3-1. GUIDE FOR IDENTIFYING A RESEARCH PROBLEM

Part 1

A. What is it in your practice that you would like to know more about? What are those things that nag you? _____

Is there an unusual pattern you've noticed in several patients that seems to be discrepant with what you've read? _____

B. Are there areas of interest that you have, from a clinical area, conceptual area, or educational experience? What are those areas that interest you most? _____

C. Out of the two above items, develop a list of simple questions about your area of interest.

D. Select one question that interests you the most. _____

E. Have you observed or read anything to help you explore the problem expressed in this question? _____

Part 2

If you had to reduce the question to two or three most important questions, what would they be? _____

Part 3

A. The following represents some common sources of information we use in nursing. Thinking over the question you have identified, consider each of the information sources and identify what type of information you might find, if any.

  1. Nursing Practice
    a. Reflection of own experience
    b. Conversation with other nurses
    c. Nursing care plans
    d. Nursing notes
    e. Observation of direct practice
    f. Historical documents

  2. Administrative Sources
    a. Quality assurance audits and reports
    b. Incident reports
    c. Twenty-four hour reports
    d. Insurance claims
    e. Change-of-shift reports

  3. Education Sources
    a. Patients and their personal support networks
    b. Education materials (eg, pamphlets)
    c. Professional education documents (eg, curriculum syllabus, test analysis)

B. Who is the focus of the question or the target group?

  1. What is the category of the person or topic in the question (eg, patient, children in day care)? _____

(Continued)

2. What are the characteristics of the person (eg, age range, diagnostic category)? _____

Part 4

What makes this study important?
Answer all that apply.

1. Because the problem occurs so often _____

2. Because the problem is severe or potentially fatal _____

3. Because the problem is amenable to intervention _____

4. Because the cost of the problem is high to people or a system _____

5. Because it's been a neglected area of study _____

Part 5

What are the benefits to be gained from studying this question.

1. Would it make nursing practice more effective? _____

2. Would patient care be improved (eg, complications reduced)? _____

3. Would answers to the question improve the efficiency of nursing practice (eg, by reducing cost, better utilization of nursing resources)? _____

4. What would happen if this question were ignored? _____

5. Other _____

Part 6

Can you identify any potential risk or harm for persons involved if you explored this question? (Consider psychological distress as well as physical harm.) _____

Part 7

Can you identify one way you might begin to explore your question (eg, conduct a survey; set up a program where some people receive a treatment and others do not; content analysis of available records)?

_____

_____

Part 8

What type of support would you need in order to develop this idea for actual study? Check all that apply.

1. Administrative _____
   a. Time off_____
   b. Clerical _____
2. Research consultation _____
   a. Design _____

(*Continued*)

b. Data analysis _____
c. Computer _____
d. Other _____
3. Tangible Support _____
  a. Money _____
  b. Equipment _____
  c. Supplies _____
  d. Library resources _____

Part 9

What other constraints can you identify that would make it difficult to carry out this study? _____

Part 10

Who can you identify that can be supportive and helpful as you carry out this research project? _____

There are available numerous indices, such as *Index Medicus,* related to the nursing literature and related disciplines. The task for the researcher is learning to be selective in the material read rather than reading everything available. The important thing is for the nurse to begin. Find an article that has to do with the general topic, even if it's not precisely on target. Additional relevant citations can often be found in the article's bibliography.

An excellent place to begin the literature review is with a review article, if one is available. Review articles may contain critiques of relevant studies and lead the researcher to the primary sources recognized by others. Published abstracts of research and other literature may also be useful in simplifying the nurse's task. A good place to begin is with the *Excerpta Medica.*

The researcher needs to develop a personal, consistent system for collecting citations and references. Once key references are noted, they tend to organize themselves without much effort. Sequences of studies begin to appear, common themes emerge, and subheadings evolve. The literature does not need to be presented in the chronological order of the citations. According to Diers (1979), the literature review should build the research questions or hypotheses of the study. The process of stating the problem, reviewing the literature, and formulating the research question or hypothesis involves feedback loops. An article may lead to changes in the problem statement; the research question may prove inadequate and require additional literature review; new literature may result in reframing the research question within the context of the problem statement. This is a dynamic process in which all the elements are constantly adjusted to maintain their fit with the other components.

Saunders, in her study on bereavement (1981), did an excellent job of identifying pertinent literature to support the questions she asked. She began her review by citing Lindeman's classic study (1944) conducted after the tragic

Coconut Grove fire in the early 40s. Saunders noted that since Lindeman's study, a number of other researchers have also categorized the behaviors and feelings of bereaved persons into phases. Common to most of the studies cited was that bereavement terminated with a recovery phase that included the formation of new relationships. While the literature substantiated that there had been an increase in knowledge about the bereavement process, Saunders was able to demonstrate that there was no general consciousness of the use of definitions of mourning, grief, and bereavement among researchers and clinicians. This process, then, gave direction to and support for her study.

One purpose of the literature review is to develop a conceptual framework for a study that identifies the major research constructs and their relationship to one another. The literature review should provoke thinking about new ways to interpret relationships among the constructs. Although Saunders' review of the literature supported the research questions she had developed, the author fell short in making explicit the conceptual framework used in her study.

DEVELOPMENT OF CONCEPTUAL FRAMEWORK

The conceptual framework provides the structure from which the investigator views the phenomena under study that are specified in the problem statement. This part of the research process is also called the "theoretical background" or "theoretical foundation." The state of existing knowledge published in the literature strongly influences how the researcher proceeds to develop the conceptual framework. The term *conceptual framework* is not to be confused with conceptual models such as Orem's self-care model (1985) or Roy's adaptation model (1984). Conceptual models influence theory generation and testing. The use of a model provides a focus that directs the questions one asks and the theories one proposes and subsequently tests. A model provides a network within which questions, theories, and data fit together and make possible the identification of needed areas of theory development (Newman, 1979).

The conceptual framework is a synthesis of some accumulated body of knowledge about the phenomena, the researcher's first-hand knowledge of the phenomena, and the available general theories that seem germane to the phenomena. The framework represents the interaction between the real world of events and the systematically accumulated body of scientific knowledge. According to Batey (1971), the conceptual framework is the researcher's image of how the phenomena he or she wants to study exist in the real world. The framework consists of three potential ideas: (1) human beings (conceptual cases); (2) behaviors or characteristics (conceptual properties of cases); and (3) ways these aspects fit together or affect each other (the relationships among properties of the cases).

By definition, the conceptual framework is analytical and is a high-level synthesis of the literature with clinical knowledge. New concepts are logically and theoretically linked. The framework develops the concepts directing the study, rather than merely presenting, listing, or identifying concepts. The development may include a historical appreciation of the roots of the concept (as Saunders implicitly developed with bereavement) as well as its empirical groundings in current research. The framework also develops the interrelatedness of the concepts. The conceptual framework is not merely presented as a repeat of previously developed ideas of others, but rather it is a careful integration of theoretical issues and areas around the problem area as the investigator chooses to view them. How the problem is characterized and what concepts and theories are pulled together to elaborate the logic and consistency of the connections between the ideas determine the value of the study's scientific contribution. For the nursing research studies discussed in this book, the following two examples are illustrated.

Bishop et al (1984) identified a straightforward and fundamental problem. They noted that uncontrolled nausea and vomiting may occur with chemotherapy; when nausea and vomiting occur, the patient's anxiety increases; the patient's anxiety may in turn contribute to poor control of the nausea and vomiting. The study was designed to test the effects of adding a medication to the antiemetic effects of another drug. The authors did not, however, present a conceptual framework. What was missing from their problem statement was the theoretical connection between anxiety and nausea and vomiting. Why was anxiety a critical mediating variable for the occurrence and control of nausea and vomiting? The answer to this question can help direct investigators to logical intervention strategies for their study and add to our knowledge of chemotherapy-related nausea and vomiting and its control and to the quality of life of patients on chemotherapy.

Lewis (1982) demonstrated this process of conceptual relationships clearly when she presented a complex and detailed problem statement about the affirmation of an individual's self-worth as it was related to personal control and quality of life. The problem statement was explicitly connected to a reinforcement paradigm containing Rotter's social learning theory and Seligman's theory of helplessness. The concepts were logically presented and led the reader to the specific hypotheses to be tested.

The ways research problems are conceptualized will differ from researcher to researcher. There are no right or wrong ways to conceptualize a problem. One may formulate different research questions by selecting different facts and ordering them on the basis of some prior notion or theory about the nature of the phenomena.

For example, studies by Lauer, Murphy, and Powers (1982) and Dodd (1984) both include problem statements related to the information needed to promote maximum understanding and acceptance of cancer among patients with this disease. Lauer, Murphy, and Powers stated the problem in exploratory and descriptive terms. They noted that patients with cancer are living longer and receiving complex treatment regimens and therefore require information to understand their illness, treatment procedures, and role in the health-care process. Patient teaching was assumed to be an integral component of health care, but there was little evidence to show if teaching done by nurses made a difference. Relevant literature citing the effects of different teaching approaches was integrated into the problem statement. The authors concluded that in order to provide patients with information to help manage health care on a long-term basis, nurses need to know how patients view their own learning needs. The researchers chose to study a fundamental question to identify the learning needs of cancer patients.

In contrast, Dodd's study (1984) was based on the assumption that people need information about their treatment, the side effects, and the management of side effects. She concluded that the types of information nurses present to patients receiving chemotherapy may influence the patient's knowledge of chemotherapy, their self-care behaviors, and their general states of effectiveness. She provided two types of information. The drug information intervention provided the names of the chemotherapeutic agents and their potential side effects. The *Side Effect Management Techniques* (SEMT) intervention was a booklet describing 44 side effects of chemotherapy and offering written information about how to manage the side effects.

STATEMENT OF PURPOSE

The specific statement of the purpose of the proposed study (Hoffman, 1969) should logically flow from the problem statement, literature review, and conceptual framework. The purpose may be written in the form of declarative statements, or questions, or in the form of hypotheses. The purpose statement narrows the broader problem statement to testable dimensions. It states exactly what the researcher plans to do to answer the questions.

Types of Questions

The form of the purpose statement will vary according to the level of inquiry. Brink and Wood (1983) have identified three levels of research that are useful in developing purpose statements (see Table 3–2). When there is little known about a research topic, the study will focus on a search for information. The purpose

TABLE 3-2. BASIC STEPS IN DEVELOPING RESEARCH QUESTIONS

Levels of Research	Stem Questions	Problem-Conceptual	Purpose Statement
Level I	"What"	Little or no literature	Declarative statement
Level II	"What is the relationship between"	Conceptual base Literature on topic but action of variables cannot be predicted	Question
Level III	"Why"	Literature on topic; action of variables can be predicted from the theory	Hypothesis

Adapted from Brink, P. & Wood, M. (1983). Basic Steps in Planning Nursing Research (2nd ed.) Monterey, CA: Wadsworth, 193.

statement begins with "What is this?" and leads to an exploration of a topic in depth. For example, the purpose statement of Lauer, Murphy, and Powers (1982) was to describe the patients' and nurses' perceptions of the learning needs of cancer patients.

Studies at the second level of inquiry ask "What's happening here?" These are questions about relationships. These questions include concepts about which the researcher has some knowledge. For example, the purpose of Lewis's (1982) study was to test whether there was a relationship between experienced personal control and quality of life in late-stage cancer patients. Questions at the second level must have a minimum of two concepts, written in such a way that they both vary. Lewis's two concepts were experienced personal control and quality of life. If the researcher can predict the exact relationship between the concepts, a level III question is needed.

Level III questions are indicated when the researcher knows which concept(s) influences the other(s) and what direction the influence will take. Questions at level III ask "Why does this relationship exist?" The answers are presented as "because" statements and include an explanation from theory or prior research. Dodd's study (1984) is an excellent example of level III questions. She presented three hypotheses to test. The first hypothesis stated that patients who received drug information, alone or in combination with other information, would have a higher rate of accurate responses to the Chemotherapy Knowledge Questionnaire after intervention than patients who do not receive the information. The two major concepts in this study were drug information and chemotherapy knowledge. With third-level questions, the researcher specifies the direction of each concept in relation to the other. The causative concept (drug information) must be capable of manipulation by the researcher. Questions at this level are developed from a theory, and the findings are discussed in relation to the conceptual framework and new knowledge contribution to the understanding of the theory.

In summary, the purpose statement will depend on the extent to which the existing body of knowledge and the researcher's creative use of first-hand knowledge can interact to permit specification of what is to be studied, its properties, and the relation among properties.

Criteria for a Good Research Question

According to Lindeman and Schantz (1982), a good research question must meet three criteria. First, the question can be answered by collecting observable evidence or empirical data; second, the question contains reference to the relationship between two or more concepts; and third, the question follows logically and consistently from what is already known about the topic.

In addition, the research question has to have significance to nursing; it must be researchable; and it must be feasible to do. The purpose of nursing research is to gain new knowledge about the discipline of nursing. Flaskerud and Halloran (1980) have identified four concepts central to the discipline of nursing: person, environment, health, and nursing. Person refers to the recipient of care; environment, to the significant others and the surroundings of the recipient of

TABLE 3-3. CANCER NURSING RESEARCH PROBLEMS OF HIGH PRIORITY

Reduce or prevent the negative effect of cancer and cancer therapy by conducting nursing research on better ways to intervene and facilitate effective management of the sequelae (eg, anorexia, cachexia, pain, discomfort, stomatitis, vomiting, etc).

Design and test support protocols for patients and families across the diagnosis and entire treatment and continuing-care spectrum to include home-care and ambulatory cancer experience phases.

Develop indicators of nursing care outcomes and nursing assessment tools. These include measures of well-being, functional status, and acuity of illness, and the concomitant nursing-care requirements according to patient age; the alteration of physiological and daily activity processes; potential recurrence of cancer; and increased risk and vulnerability.

Promote and ensure effective professional decision making by developing (1) better communication between the nurse oncologist and the physician oncologist; (2) efficient information transfer of what is state-of-the-art and effective technology (eg, pain management, palliative care) from research to practice; and (3) mutual treatment goal setting by patients, families, nurses, and physicians.

Enhance the health protective behavior of patients by finding better ways for the nursing-care delivery system to be responsive to patient and family care, in particular, as inpatient care interfaces with outpatient care. This includes follow-up studies to assess the quality of life of survivors.

care, as well as to the setting in which nursing care occurs; health, to the wellness or illness state of the recipient; and nursing, to the actions taken by nurses. They recommended that research in clinical nursing include one or more of these four central concepts.

In the past, speciality groups including both clinicians and researchers have met to identify specific areas for nursing research in cancer patient management. In 1984, five important target areas were identified for cancer nursing research[1]. These areas are presented in Table 3-3. One method of testing whether a research question is significant is to judge whether the question fits within the content areas recommended by experts.

RELATIONSHIPS OF RESEARCH QUESTION
TO NURSING THEORY

Theory directs research and research findings shape the development of theory (Fawcett, 1978). The growth of knowledge about nursing depends on an interac-

[1]On July 26, 1984, an oncology nursing research workshop was held under the auspices of the Community Oncology and Rehabilitation Branch of the National Cancer Institute's Division of Cancer Prevention and Control. Nurse consultants, NCI staff, and guests from National Institute of Health and the Division of Nursing, Public Health Service, DDHS met to discuss research priorities for oncology nursing in the treatment, rehabilitation, and continuing care of cancer patients.

tion between the concrete realities and pragmatic domains of nursing and the abstract world of those interrelated propositions known as theories. Theories are valuable because they describe, explain, and predict, at a variety of levels, the world or nature, including human behavior in health and illness (Benoliel, 1977). When a study is directed by a specific theory, findings should effect any needed modifications in the theory. These modifications are then tested in future research endeavors. Thus, theory is developed from successive tests and revisions as new findings are uncovered. The ultimate test of a nursing theory is its pragmatism. The utility and significance of a nursing theory are determined by its ability to enable the clinician to control or alter the major concepts and conditions specified by the theory to bring about the most effective outcomes for the recipients of nursing care.

SUMMARY

In this chapter, the basic steps for developing a research question were presented. The steps included in the conceptual phase of research are: the identification of the research problem, the selection of a researchable problem, the review of the literature, the development of the conceptual framework, and the statement of purpose. The conceptual phase identifies the dimensions of knowledge that bear on the phenomena of interest and describes the researcher's image of how those phenomena operate or exist in the empirical world. The conceptual phase guides the researcher to the decisions that .direct the substance and the procedures of data production, analysis, and interpretation.

Therefore, the conceptual phase may be regarded as the most challenging part of the research process. It provides opportunities for creative thinkers to combine theoretical perspectives and clinical insights into elegant research questions out of which new understandings can emerge to benefit nursing and the recipients of nursing care.

REFERENCES

Batey, M. (1971). Conceptualizing the research project. *Nursing Research, 20*(4), 296–301.

Batey, M. (1977). Conceptualization: Knowledge and logic guiding empirical research. *Nursing Research, 26*(5), 324–329.

Benoliel, J. (1977). The interaction between theory and research. *Nursing Outlook, 25*(2), 108–113.

Benner, P., & Wrubel, J. (1982). Skilled clinical knowledge: The value of perceptual awareness, part 1. *Journal of Nursing Administration, 12*(5), 11–14.

Benner, P. (1984). *From novice to expert: Excellence and power in clinical nursing practice.* Menlo Park, CA: Addison-Wesley.

Bishop, J., Olver, I.N., Wolf, M., et al (1984). Lorazepam: A randomized, double-blind, crossover study of a new antiemetic in patients receiving cytotoxic chemotherapy and prochlorperazine. *Journal of Clinical Oncology, 2*(6), 691–695.

Brink, P., & Wood, J. (1983). *Basic steps in planning nursing research, from question to proposal.* 2nd Edition. Monterey, CA: Jones and Bartlett.

Diers, D. (1979). *Research in nursing practice.* Philadelphia: Lippincott.

Dodd, M. (1984). Measuring informational intervention for chemotherapy knowledge and self-care behavior. *Research in Nursing and Health, 7*(1), 43–50.

Fawcett, J. (1978). Practice oriented theory: The relationship between theory and research: A double helix. *Advances in Nursing Science, 1*(5), 49–62.

Flaskerud, J.H., & Halloran, E.J. (1980). Areas of agreement in nursing theory development. *Advances in Nursing Science, 3*(1), 1–7.

Fleming, J. (1984). Selecting a clinical nursing problem for research. *Image, 16*(1), 62–64.

Hoffman, K. (1969). Problem identification and the research design. In M. Batey (Ed.), *Communicating Nursing Research* (5–11). Boulder, CO: Western Interstate Commission for Higher Education.

Lauer, P., Murphy, S., Powers, M. (1982). Learning needs of cancer patients: A comparison of nurse and patient perceptions. *Nursing Research, 31*(1), 11–16.

Lewis, F.M. (1982). Experienced personal control and quality of life in late-stage cancer patients. *Nursing Research, 31*(2), 113–119.

Lindeman, C., & Schantz, D. (1982). The research question. *Journal of Nursing Administration, 12*(1), 6–10.

Lindemann, E. (1944). Symptomatology and management of acute grief. *American Journal of Psychiatry, 101*(July), 141–148.

Lindsey, A. (1983). Research: The problem and the purpose. *Oncology Nursing Forum, 10*(3), 97–98.

McCorkle, R. (1974). Effects of touch on seriously-ill patients. *Nursing Research, 23*(2), 125–132.

Newman, M.A. (1979). *Theory development in nursing.* Philadelphia: Davis.

Orem, D. (1985). *Nursing: Concepts of practice.* (3rd ed.). New York: McGraw-Hill.

Padilla, G. (1979). Incorporating research in service setting. *Journal of Nursing Administration, 9*(1), 44–49.

Padilla, G., Baker, V., Dolan, V. (1977). Interacting with dying patients. In M. Batey (Ed.), *Communicating Nursing Research* (101–114). Boulder, CO: Western Interstate Commission for Higher Education.

Rotter, J. (1964). *Clinical psychology.* Englewood Cliffs, NJ: Prentice-Hall.

Roy, C. (1984). *Introduction to nursing: An adaptation model.* Englewood Cliffs, NJ: Prentice-Hall.

Saunders, J. (1981). A process of bereavement resolution: Uncoupled identity. *Western Journal of Nursing Research, 3*(Fall), 319–336.

Schantz, D., & Lindeman, C. (1982). Reading a research article. *Journal of Nursing Administration, 12*(3) 30–33.

Seligman, M. (1975). *Helplessness: On depression, development, and death.* San Francisco: Freeman.

Valiga, T., & Mermel, V. (1985). Formulating the research question. *Topics in Clinical Nursing, 7*(2) 1–14.

Wilson, H.S. (1985). *Research in nursing.* Menlo Park, CA: Addison-Wesley.

CHAPTER 4

Development of the Theoretical Framework

Eleanor Saltzer

This chapter is dedicated to my son David, through whom I have learned more about cancer and chemotherapy than I ever wanted to know about the subjects, and also to my husband, Gene, and my daughter Becky, who have shared in the experience.

Although the theoretical background for cancer nursing research can be derived from several scientific disciplines, such as biology, physiology, sociology, medicine, and others; the emphasis in this chapter will be primarily on psychosocial frameworks, with occasional mention of frameworks derived from other fields, such as physiology or public health. It should be made clear from the outset that this chapter is not intended to be an exhaustive review of all possible theoretical frameworks for cancer nursing research. Rather, the chapter is designed to illustrate the use of various theoretical frameworks by presenting a collection of *selected* theories that are currently potentially useful to nurses for research about cancer. One final introductory comment is in order. Nurse scholars as well as social scientists have generated the frameworks that this chapter will highlight. The use of theories developed by nurses as well as by scientists in other fields adds richness and variety to the texture of oncology nursing research, in addition to broadening the field of ideas to be explored.

RESEARCH TERMS RELATED TO THEORETICAL FRAMEWORKS

The development of theory is the motivation for all research, including research in nursing. A *theory* is a declaration of interrelated propositions about observed phenomena that has been verified to some degree. From a research perspective, propositions are statements to be upheld or problems to be solved. Relationships express how various propositions are connected to each other. Theories are developed and used to explain or interpret observations. Theories are built upon truths or doctrines on which other conclusions are based. These truths or doctrines are called *principles*.

The *theoretical framework* refers to the various theories that may be used in the development of a study. A theoretical framework may be thought of as the point of departure for a specific investigation. Usually the particular theoretical framework governing a study is explained in the initial review-of-the-literature portion of a research proposal or report.

For instance, Lewis (1982) (*see* Appendix) the research question is developed from two basic theories in the field of social science. The first theory is Rotter's social learning theory (Rotter, 1954, 1966, 1974), in which certain propositions about motivation for behavior and learning are set forth. Lewis incorporates ideas derived from social learning theory about internal versus external "locus of control." An individual with internal locus of control beliefs expects that he or she is responsible for the outcomes of actions, whereas a person with external locus of control beliefs expects that outcomes are governed by luck, fate, or chance. Lewis combines these ideas with questions raised by another social science theory known as the theory of "learned helplessness" (Seligman, 1975). The theory of learned helplessness offers an explanation for learning behaviors that indicate that an individual doubts voluntary action will achieve desired outcomes.

Both the social learning theory and the theory of learned helplessness represent certain propositions about relationships that have been examined in research about motivation, learning, and behavior. However, in combining the theories of social learning and learned helplessness, Lewis extends her ideas and develops a unique arrangement of propositions for the particular research study she devised on experienced personal control and quality of life in late-stage cancer patients.

In summary, a theory is one interrelated set of principles, relationships, propositions, and explanations, whereas a theoretical framework is broader and may refer to the structural arrangement of ideas drawing on multiple discrete theories to guide research. Simply stated, the theoretical framework is the frame of reference for a specific research project. As such, the framework guides the research, establishes the relationships between the variables studied, and provides the basis for the hypotheses or questions examined in the research. However, the theoretical framework also provides the basis for the interpretation of the results of a study. When the data have been collected and analyzed, the researcher must ask the question, how do the findings relate to the original framework of the study. Are the findings consistent with the initial predictions? If not, then why not?

Theoretical frameworks are also important for generating theory as in the "grounded theory approach" (Glaser & Strauss, 1967). In the case of qualitative research, the use of the theoretical framework is essential for the analysis phase of a descriptive study. The theoretical framework guides the interpretation of observations and enhances the generalizability of findings (Artinian, 1982). Several research terms related to "theoretical framework" are paradigm, concept, variable, conceptual map, hypothesis, research model, and causal model.

COMMON THEORETICAL FRAMEWORKS IN CANCER NURSING RESEARCH

Theoretical frameworks used in cancer nursing research are influenced by the practical goal of appropriate nursing intervention. Using public health terminology, we can categorize the overall goal of cancer nursing intervention into interventions directed toward various levels of prevention (Burns, 1982). Primary prevention refers to preventing the development of a disease. This can be accomplished either by altering the environment or by changing characteristics of individuals so they will no longer be susceptible to a disease. Secondary prevention refers to the early diagnosis and treatment of the disease. Finally, tertiary prevention refers to minimizing the consequences of a disease through rehabilitation or adjustment after treatment for a disease. For the purposes of this chapter, we will organize the discussion of theoretical frameworks around the level of prevention toward which the theory is principally directed.

PRIMARY PREVENTION: REDUCING THE RISK OF DISEASE

Primary prevention in cancer research examines risk factors of individuals, environmental risks, occupational risks, and studies of the general epidemiology of cancer to identify these risks (Holland & Karhausen, 1979). Nursing research in the area of primary prevention is not limited to studies of individuals. Primary prevention nursing research may be community-wide, as in the work of McLaughlin (1982), who has identified a model of community health programs in order to promote health and thereby eliminate potential risk factors for cancer. Occupational health nursing research may examine health and safety standards in the workplace to limit exposure to carcinogens, such as asbestos. Primary prevention research by nurses may even extend to the political arena, as in the area of public policy research to examine the economic and legislative issues related to elimination of potential carcinogens from the environment (Burns, 1982).

In general, categories of cancer nursing research and primary prevention, the theoretical frameworks deal with independent variables that affect the incidence of disease and dependent variables that evaluate the presence or absence of malignancy. Researchers approaching studies of cancer from a primary preventive point of view are interested in examining the complex mechanisms that interact between community or individual behavior and the development of cancer.

Strategies for Interventions to Promote Health

Health-related behaviors are appropriate preventive and curative actions performed by individuals to influence their own health. Motivating people to perform appropriate preventive and curative actions is the major goal of health education (Leventhal, Safer, & Panagis, 1983). Several theoretical frameworks have been useful in the study of strategies to design interventions for cancer prevention through the promotion of health-related behaviors.

Locus of Control and Health. Locus of control (Rotter, 1966) is one category of expectancy beliefs derived from the general expectancy–value theory of motivation (Atkinson, 1964). Expectancy–value theories all share the proposition that the motivation for performing a given behavior is a function of the expectancy about the outcome of the behavior multiplied by the value of the outcome. This proposition is expressed by the formula:

$$m = e \times v$$

in which m = motivation, e = expectancy, and v = value.

The concept, also known as a construct, of internal–external locus of control relates to expectancies about the outcomes of action (Lefcourt, 1981, 1982; Phares, 1976; Rotter, 1966). Locus of control is viewed as a continuum of expectancy beliefs ranging from extremely internal to extremely external expectancies.

It has been argued that locus of control does not really refer to one dimension but may actually incorporate separate beliefs about the degree to which events are under personal control, chance control, or control by powerful others (Levenson, 1973, 1974). Rotter (1974) has argued that for specific behaviors and situations it may be more appropriate to measure specific internal–external locus of control expectancies rather than one generalized belief tapped by Rotter's (1966) Internal–External (I–E) scale and similar measures. It has been demonstrated that internals and externals differ in their responsiveness to forms of social influence (Phares, 1976). In reviewing the locus-of-control literature, Lefcourt (1982) concludes that externals show greater conformity and are less willing to resist social pressures than internals.

Among the possible consequences of a belief in external control by powerful others may be the development of behavior directed at appeasing or pleasing those who are in control. If one cannot influence the perceived social environment directly, then perhaps one can gain the favor of those who are perceived to control the social environment. Those who believe the world is too difficult for them to control may attempt to imitate or please other people who are perceived to be more successful. Thus, a possible outcome of an external locus of control orientation may be a greater motivation to behave in a way that is responsive to perceived social pressures in the environment.

Locus of control beliefs have been widely researched in relation to health behaviors. Wallston and Wallston (1978) conclude that, in general, internality is associated with good health. Consequently, they advocate that health-care professionals develop techniques to train people to be more internally motivated with respect to health. However, whether it is always preferable to be internal with respect to health has been questioned by Saltzer and Saltzer (1987), who suggest that further research should identify those specific health situations in which internality or externality represents successful coping.

Rotter (1974) states that in specific situations, where each slight increment in predictability may have important consequences, scales measuring specific expectancies relevant to the situation might be more useful than the general I-E scale. The need for specific measures of health-related locus-of-control expectancies exists in the area of health research because increased predictability may have practical advantages for health care.

For this reason, researchers in health behavior developed specific health locus-of-control measures. Wallston and Wallston developed and validated a Health Locus of Control (HLC) Scale (Wallston et al, 1976) and later published the Multidimensional Health Locus of Control (MHLC) Scales (Wallston, Wallston, & DeVellis, 1978).

The MHLC Scales incorporate concepts of the HLC Scale, but there are three specific scales measuring the belief that health is internally controlled, externally controlled by powerful others, or externally controlled by chance. Alagna and Reddy (1984) used the MHLC Scales to measure variance in the performance of breast self-examination. Belief in powerful others health locus of control and belief in chance health locus of control were both negatively related to proficient breast self-examination; whereas belief in internal health locus of control was not significantly correlated with breast self-examination behaviors. The strongest positive predictor of proficient breast self-examination behaviors was confidence in the efficacy of breast self-examination to detect tumors. For future research on locus of control and health, there may also be a need for additional specific measures of locus of control for various other clinical conditions as an aid to nursing research and practice.

The Health Belief Model. The Health Belief Model (HBM) has been specifically formulated for the prediction of health-related behaviors (Rosenstock, 1966). The underlying assumptions of the HBM are heavily invested in a "rational" view of man. The model's purpose is to predict health behaviors. However, another function of the HBM is to identify important areas for interventions directed toward the promotion of positive health-related actions (Rosenstock & Kirscht, 1974). The HBM was developed by public health experts whose academic roots were in the field of social psychology (Rosenstock, 1974). Moreover, like the construct of locus of control, formulation of the model was strongly influenced by expectancy–value theories of motivation (Maiman & Becker, 1974).

The HBM has evolved from Rosenstock's first description of it in the literature (Becker & Maiman, 1975; Janz & Becker, 1984). A comprehensive statement of the HBM (Becker et al, 1977) consists of a dependent variable and two groups of independent variables. The dependent variable is the likelihood of compliance with either preventive health recommendations or prescribed regimens. The likelihood of compliance is influenced by the two groups of predictor variables consisting of "readiness" variables and "modifying" variables, which reciprocally act upon each other in addition to influencing the dependent variable of "compliance."

Readiness to undertake recommended compliance behavior is further subdivided into the categories of motivations, perceived threat posed by illnesses or conditions, and perceived probability that compliant behavior will reduce the threat. The readiness component of the model is composed entirely of cognitions. It incorporates expectancy–value beliefs. The value is measured by the motivations and by the perceived threat posed by illnesses or conditions, whereas expectancies are measured by the perceived probability that compliant behavior will reduce the threat (Maiman & Becker, 1974).

The modifying factors consist of variables that have been found through prior research to be associated with health behaviors. One group of modifying factors consists of demographic and social variables including age, sex, race, marital status, income, and education. A second group of modifying factors includes perceived structural factors, which were called "perceived barriers" in Rosenstock's earlier version of the HBM (1966). Structural factors consist of perceptions of the regimen's safety, complexity, cost, accessibility, duration, and difficulty. Other modifying factors are attitudes and interpersonal interactions. The final group of this category of variables contains the enabling factors. These consist of prior experience with the health action, condition, or regimen, and also the extent of family problems (Becker et al, 1977).

The Theory of Reasoned Action. The theory of reasoned action (Ajzen & Fishbein, 1980) is a model of behavioral intentions (Fishbein & Ajzen, 1975) that, like the construct of locus of control and the Health Belief Model, is formulated in expectancy–value terms (Atkinson, 1964). This theory, however, emphasizes the way in which expectancy values influence the intention to perform a given behavior. The model expresses the relationship between attitudes, behavioral intentions, and behavior by proposing that there are two immediate or proximal determinants of behavior consisting of (1) the individual's personal attitude toward the behavior; and (2) the external social norms (ie, what important others expect the person to do with respect to the behavior in question). Behavioral intentions, moreover, are proposed to be highly predictive of actual behavior.

Fishbein & Ajzen (1975) argue that personal attitudes and perceived social pressures are the only two factors that directly determine intentions to perform a given behavior. Variables outside the model, such as personality characteristics, are said to affect behavioral intentions only indirectly by influencing the personal attitudinal component, the social normative component, or the relative weights of the two components.

The evidence from research investigations in both laboratory and natural situations supports the assumption that behavioral intentions can be highly predictive of and even approximately equivalent to actual behavior. The theory of reasoned action is useful for providing specific information about which specific attitudes and social pressures influence health-related behavior.

Self-Efficacy Theory. Self-efficacy is "the conviction that one can successfully execute the behavior required to produce the outcomes" (Bandura, 1977, p. 193). Individuals' self-efficacy beliefs relate to their perceptions of their own skills for performing given behaviors. Moreover, self-efficacy expectations are concerned with a person's sense of personal mastery. Activity choices and the selection of behavior settings are influenced by efficacy expectations, as well as by incentives or perceived values and by actual abilities. People tend to avoid activities for which they lack competence and also tend to avoid threatening situations.

Furthermore, self-efficacy expectations influence effort and persistency in the face of obstacles. Successful coping results from stronger efficacy expectations, and at the same time greater persistence at difficult tasks may lead to heightened feelings of self-efficacy.

Condiotte and Lichtenstein (1981) and McIntyre, Lichtenstein, and Mermelstein (1983) have used a framework of self-efficacy theory to study smoking cessation. Moreover, Alagna and Reddy (1984) in their study of breast self-examination, while not specifically using Bandura's format, found that perceived self-efficacy was the most significant predictor of proficiency in breast self-examination. In fact, for the Alagna and Reddy study, self-efficacy was a stronger predictor than multidimensional health locus of control beliefs or the Health Belief Model.

Communications to Promote Health. Regardless of the theoretical framework used to study the determinants of health-related behaviors, the purpose of these types of investigations is to develop effective communication methods for the promotion of health behaviors. We will now examine some of the general findings of research about communication techniques designed to promote preventive health behaviors. Studies on public health communication may look at mass communication or communication in small groups or individual communication as Kegeles (1983) points out. It is well established that mass communication can successfully reach a health population. Appropriate communication may be successful in persuading people to follow health-related behaviors.

One extensive line of research about communication and health has been the work of Leventhal (1970). Leventhal is concerned about whether fear appeals will influence behavior. The main finding of Leventhal's research is that fear associated with health communication will influence behavior if there is a specific action to be taken associated with the fear appeal. Global fear appeals do not necessarily influence subsequent behavior; and, in fact, if the fear appeals are too high, they may result in denial of the necessity of taking action.

Leventhal has continued to expand and modify his views on communication. His earlier research viewed subjects as passive recipients of information; whereas his more recent research has focused on individuals as active processors of information.

In summary, Green (1970), a health educator, states that the main goals of health education in the cancer program are to obtain individual, voluntary health actions. These actions must also take place without any external public sanctions. In other words, the individual must voluntarily participate in the appropriate health behaviors. In the area of cancer education, Green states that mass communication is the most frequently used method.

Stress, Social Support, and the Onset of Cancer

The second major aspect in the study of primary prevention of cancer examines those factors that increase or decrease the likelihood that an individual may develop cancer. Such studies often result from social epidemiologic investigations, trying to link together personality or situational variables that relate to the onset of cancer. Two important factors are stress and social support.

Stress and the Etiology of Cancer. Studies of human beings, as well as animals, have indicated that there may be a link between stress and the development of cancer (Anisman & Zacharko, 1983; Bieliauskas, 1983). However, as Cohen and Lazarus (1979) point out, the research evidence that connects stress to the etiology of cancer is not clearly defined. The specific biological link between stress and the etiology of cancer has yet to be completely elucidated. According to Burns (1982), the theories that connect stress with the onset of cancer usually hypothesize failure of an aspect of the immune system, or a proliferation of hormones resulting from stress that somehow induces the development of tumors, or a combination of both factors. The importance of studying stress in connection with the primary prevention of cancer is ultimately to promote stress reduction behaviors as a method of cancer prevention.

In the absence of evidence for specific biological links between stress and cancer, there have evolved several typical patterns of research that relate stress to the etiology of cancer. One theoretical framework examines stressful life events and their impact on the onset of cancer. A second theoretical framework examines behaviors that are related to stress and that subsequently promote the onset of cancer. Another approach is to examine personality variables in relation to levels of chronic stress. Finally, there are those studies that examine immunocompetence and the etiology of cancer.

Stressful Life Events. Building upon the work of Selye (1956), who postulated a "general adaptation syndrome," two researchers, Holmes and Rahe (1967), developed a Social Readjustment Rating Scale (SRRS). This scale is based upon the premise that change in life is critical to health and that normative ratings established by judges can determine the amount of adjustment required by an individual. Moreover, the scale assumes that a given life event requires the same amount of adjustment for different people, and finally, that different types of events can be clustered together to develop a score of adjustment requirement. After the publication of the Social Readjustment Rating Scale, many researchers began to study the correlation of scores on the scale with the onset of disease. This type of research has been dubbed "stressful life events" research and is well summarized in the book of the same name by Dohrenwend and Dohrenwend (1974).

There are methodological problems in the study of stressful life events and the onset of illness. First of all, the stressful life events research is correlational; therefore, one can only establish that there is a relationship between stressful life events scores and the development of disease. This does not necessarily support a causal argument. Second, the SRRS assumes that all life events, whether they are positive or negative life events, have the same impact upon an illness. Some researchers have questioned whether negative life events, such as the loss of a job, have a greater impact upon an individual than a positive life event, such as a promotion to a new job. Both events may be stressful but the quality of the stress may vary and, therefore, may have a differing impact upon an individual. Third, some life events are difficult to define to the outside researcher. Finally, the stressful life events research is not specific; scores on the scale do not predict the onset of a specific type of illness or even the onset of cancers in general, but rather point to a greater likelihood of the development of *some* type of illness, such as heart disease, gastrointestinal disorders, upper respiratory infections, accidents, or cancer. Therefore, using the Social Readjustment Rating Scale alone is not sufficient to predict the development of a specific tumor.

Behavior and Stress. Studies have examined the relationships of certain behaviors to stress and, in particular, where those behaviors are known to be related to cancer. For example, smoking may be viewed as a behavior that is a response to stress and thus is related to the etiology of cancer. An example of this type of research can be found in the study of occupational stress by Conway, et al (1981). This study examines the impact of occupational stress on self-reported consumption of cigarettes, coffee, and alcohol. The implication is that if stress causes excessive smoking, this behavioral response may be related to the onset of lung cancer.

Personality and Stress. Cohen and Lazarus (1979) review numerous studies that relate various personality types to the development of cancer. For example, personality variables implicated in the development of cancer include the inability to express hostile feelings and emotion, personalities who are anally fixated, individuals who extensively use repression and denial as defense mechanisms, individuals who are emotional and extroverted, or alternatively individuals who are introverted, individuals who report less closeness to parents, and individuals who have suffered a significant loss or separation.

Kobasa (1982) has postulated a general personality trait that protects against illness. This personality trait Kobasa has designated the "hardy personality." Kobasa postulates that "hardiness" mediates between the impact of stressful life events and the number and severity of illness reports. The three basic concepts of Kobasa's hardiness trait derive from the philosophy of existentialism. These traits are (1) commitments that involve self-esteem, personal competence, and a sense of community; (2) control, which is the tendency to believe and act as though one can influence the outcome of events; and (3) challenge, which is based on the belief that change is normal in life. Kobasa has demonstrated in several studies that the personality variable of hardiness is related to the avoidance of disease. Again, as with the research on stressful life events, Kobasa's research is not disease-specific; it merely shows a personality trait that is related to health. However, examining personality variables that relate to a lower incidence of disease is a departure from more traditional correlational studies that examine personality variables as deficits that promote disease.

Immunocompetence, Endocrinology, and the Etiology of Cancer. While this chapter primarily emphasizes sociopsychological theoretical frameworks, an important avenue of physiological research must be mentioned in relation to stress—research on immunocompetence. Burns (1982) and the American Cancer Society (1981) summarize the theories related to immune system failure and the onset of cancer. This avenue of research endeavors to find the specific biological connections between stress and cancer. Studies of immunocompetence and the etiology of cancer have used both animal and human models and have noted a relationship between immunosuppressive drugs and the development of certain tumors as well as immunosuppression and the reduction of the growth of certain specific tumors. Closely related are studies of the endocrine system and the onset of or resistence to tumor growth. The complexity of the relationship between the immune system, the endocrine system, and the development of tumors remains to be completely explored; however, this certainly is an essential area of research for refining our understanding of the biological basis of the development of cancer. Finding the physiological connection between perceived stress and the development of cancer will significantly enhance preventive efforts to the reduction of stress.

Social Support and the Prevention of Disease. Social support is a concept that refers to the ways in which social relationships presumably protect people from the harmful effects of stress (Wortman, 1984). Much research has suggested that social support somehow "innoculates" people from the negative effects of stress (Janis, 1983; Wortman, 1984). However, according to Wortman, there is little information known about the underlying mechanisms, if any, by which social support actually influences health outcomes. Despite many conceptual and methodological issues related to the study of social support, it continues to be a currently popular variable that apparently mediates between stress and health (Wortman, 1984).

Janis (1983) proposes that social support is a significant variable for adherence to stressful decisions. Examples that Janis uses to indicate his point of view are the success of programs offering counseling for smoking cessation or weight control. Many individuals are able successfully to avoid the undesired behaviors of smoking or overeating while regularly meeting with a counselor. However, once the counseling is ended, the rate of relapse to the old behaviors is high within one or two months following cessation of the counseling.

Three critical phases determine the degree to which counselors can be change agents: building up of referent power, using referent power, and retaining referent power after contact ends and promoting internalization. The significance of Janis' work on counseling is that he emphasizes that social support intervenes to influence adherence to stressful decisions or behaviors that in fact promote health.

SECONDARY PREVENTION: DIAGNOSIS AND TREATMENT

Secondary prevention refers to the diagnosis and treatment of disease. For this portion of the chapter we will examine those theoretical frameworks relating to nursing care that facilitates seeking of a medical diagnosis of cancer as well as nursing care for the treatment of patients with cancer.

The approach to the section on the diagnosis of cancer will be to examine patient variables that lead to patients' pursuit of a medical diagnosis rather than to review the pathophysiologic techniques for confirming a particular medical diagnosis. Two main theoretical frameworks focus on the steps leading to the diagnosis of illness. The first framework deals with how an individual recognizes that physical symptoms present may actually be illness. Closely related is the study of how one determines that recognized physical symptoms require health-related actions.

The area of secondary prevention referring to diagnosis and treatment for illness focuses on research about nursing care of the cancer patient in an acute-care facility. In fact, several of the special nursing care needs of oncology patients discussed in this section may also apply to the oncology patient at home and hence are also applicable to nursing practice in an outpatient, public health, or visiting nurse setting.

Diagnosis of Cancer

Recognition of Physical Symptoms as Illness. Pennebaker (1982) has extensively examined the psychology of physical symptoms. He has cited several factors that influence the interpretation of physical sensations: attention, interpretive sets, and moods. The focusing of attention onto bodily states has been found to increase symptom reporting, while distraction reduces symptom reporting, according to Pennebacker and Skelton (1978).

The interpretive set reflects whether the subject perceives the sensation as positive or negative. Pain is assumed by Pennebaker and Skelton (1978) to be a negative physical sensation. However, nonpainful sensation, for example, a racing heartbeat, may have ambiguous interpretations.

Moods have also been found by Pennebaker and Skelton (1978) to be associated with levels of symptom reporting; negative moods relate to higher levels of symptom reports. The direction of the correlational data between mood and symptom reports has not been resolved at present. That is, do negative moods cause perceptions of more symptoms, or does the presence of physical symptoms lead to negative moods? Perhaps moods and physical symptoms interact to exacerbate one another. Pennebaker and Skelton hypothesize that moods may function as a type of interpretive set for evaluating physical sensations.

Rodin (1978) has proposed that "availability" is another factor that influences the interpretation of physical sensations. The availability hypothesis states that judgments about the probability of being affected by a given disease depend to an extent upon which images of that disease are in the minds of people who think about the disease. Availability of disease images may be influenced by news reports of celebrities having a particular disorder. Moreover, availability may be influenced by the unique history of the individual. That is, if the person has, for example, been closely associated with a friend or relative having a given disease. People may tend to underestimate the likelihood of developing diseases with which they are unfamiliar but may tend to overestimate the likelihood of developing a disease that is close to the individual's own experience or that has received much publicity.

The mass media efforts to educate the public on cancer, plus the widespread presence of cancer, may make this disorder one of the more available diagnoses that people consider when they experience a physical symptom. An interesting area of research would be to explore the frequency with which individuals interpret perceived physical sensations as potentially being cancer. A factor also related to these interpretations is the issue of fear and denial of a potential diagnosis. An interesting comparison could be made by examining what is the stronger motivation for seeking medical care: concern that physical symptoms may be caused by cancer and thereby leading to early treatment seeking or fear of a dreaded disease leading to denial and avoidance of medical treatment.

Personal Attributions of Illness.   Attribution theory is the study of the interpretations that individuals place upon experiences they have or observe (Heider, 1958; Jones & Davis, 1965; Kelley, 1967). Researchers have proposed that a fruitful approach to the study of health-related behaviors is to understand how people interpret and give significance to the experiences they have. This line of investigation uses the techniques of attribution theory (Mechanic, 1975; Rodin, 1978). Physical symptoms are perceived as contributing to illness when usual behavior is disrupted by the symptoms (Mechanic, 1975). Recognizing that there may be individual differences in the degree to which symptoms disrupt usual functioning, Mechanic asserts that when symptoms reach the point of interfering with usual functioning, people are more likely to take health-related actions.

Further, Mechanic (1972) found that when people experience changes in usual functioning, they attempt to test hypotheses about the causes and seriousness of their symptoms. The subsequent attributions affect the perceived meaning of the symptoms and the ensuing courses of action.

The cognitive interpretations given to perceived bodily states; how symptoms are perceived as illnesses by individuals; and the demographic, social-structural, cultural, and personality variables that affect health-care use all influence the extent to which individuals will seek a medical diagnosis for a perceived physical symptom. Rodin (1978) has concluded that individual attributions of causality have a profound impact on many aspects of health-related behavior. Future research is needed to understand those aspects of attributions and interpretations of physical symptoms that will motivate individuals to seek a confirmed medical diagnosis that may result in the negative information that cancer is present.

Research on Nursing Care of Patients Undergoing Cancer Treatment

The main emphasis of nursing actions is to provide care and comfort measures for patients who are otherwise diseased or disabled as a result of an illness and related medical intervention (Riehl & Roy, 1980). Oncology nursing is especially involved with administering care-related measures (American Cancer Society, 1981; Anderson, 1982; Burns, 1982; Klagsbrun, 1970) because the rigorous principal ingredients of cancer therapy are either surgery, chemotherapy, or radiation therapy, used alone or in some combination with each other. All these major treatment programs involve extended periods of discomfort as a result of the therapy. It is during this time that nursing care can most assist to alleviate many of the major consequences of these three principal medical intervention modalities. Research on the nursing care of patients undergoing cancer treatment may generally focus on the application of nursing conceptual models to nursing intervention or may focus specifically on individual nursing diagnoses related to cancer patient care.

Nursing Conceptual Models. Nursing models govern nursing actions in that the way a nurse views practice will determine what appropriate items of patient care will be assessed and what interventions will be applied best to provide comfort and promote recovery for a given patient. Excellent reviews of various developed nursing models are provided by Riehl and Roy (1980) and Fawcett (1984). The principal purpose of nursing conceptual models is to distinguish nursing actions that are independent and unique to the practice of nursing from other related actions of the health professions.

The study of nursing conceptual models may provide the theoretical basis for cancer nursing research. For example, Derdiarian (1983) and Derdiarian and Forsythe (1983) developed an instrument to study cancer patients based upon the behavioral systems model for nursing developed by Johnson (1959) and embellished in the work by Auger (1976). Dodd (1984a, 1984b) has developed an avenue of research with oncology patients using Orem's (1980) nursing concept of self-care. An article by Dodd (1984a) is summarized in the appendix. These reports are all excellent examples of the use of a particular nursing model as it is applied to the care of the cancer patient.

The current term used to describe the identification of independent nursing care problems is nursing diagnosis (Campbell, 1984; Carpenito, 1983, 1984; Kim, McFarland, & McLane, 1984). Over time, nursing research may tend to identify and enlarge the concept of nursing diagnosis. Research on nursing diagnosis has much to accomplish. To facilitate the development of this concept for nursing practice and research, we will review several special nursing care problems of hospitalized oncology patients from the framework of nursing diagnosis. The nursing theoretical frameworks that are pertinent to care of patients undergoing cancer therapy include anxiety and fear, anorexia, nausea and vomiting, pain, knowledge deficits, body image, disturbances, grieving, loss of personal control, coping, adherence to prescribed regimens, and social support. The theories that may elucidate the study of the nursing diagnoses presented herein are selective in that they focus primarily, but not exclusively, on psychological and sociological perspectives and interventions.

Anxiety and Fear: The Crisis of the Diagnosis of Cancer. Anxiety and fear are two separate nursing diagnoses according to present classification standards (Carpenito, 1983, 1984; Kim, McFarland, & McLane, 1984). However, anxiety and fear may both be present in the same individual at the same time (Carpenito, 1983, 1984). The clinical distinctions between anxiety and fear are that anxiety relates to those feelings of apprehension and uneasiness that are in response to a vague, nonspecific threat; whereas fear describes those same feelings and experiences in relation to an identifiable stimulus that is perceived as dangerous. Anxiety and fear may relate to the diagnosis of cancer or to concerns about the specific treatments including surgery, chemotherapy, or radiation therapy (Anderson, et al, 1984).

Experts in the field of health care agree that for many individuals the knowledge that one has an illness diagnosed as cancer is a form of life crisis (American Cancer Society, 1981; Burns, 1982; Germino, 1982; Horan, 1982; and Moos & Tsu, 1977). Because of the severe personal, social, and societal consequences of the disease of cancer, individuals have a great fear of receiving this diagnosis. Interventions by the nursing staff to provide supportive mechanisms can be vital to the individual who is overcoming both physical symptoms and debilitation, disruption of life, fear of death, and the physical discomforts related to medical interventions for the treatment of cancer.

Nursing research in relation to the crisis of the diagnosis of cancer can center on patient responses and appropriate nursing crisis intervention techniques for oncology patients and their families. For example, Frank-Stromborg, et al, (1984) have described several themes most frequently cited by oncology patients as their initial feelings after being diagnosed as having cancer. They are positive attitudes, shock, fear or disbelief, anger, depression, or hopelessness, did not want to think about it, amputation of the future, renewed faith, feeling of doom, and multiple reactions combining several themes at the same time. As a result of their research, Frank-Stromborg et al recommend that nurses assess which of these feelings patients are experiencing before implementing patient education, referrals, or psychosocial support.

The crisis of the diagnosis of cancer has an impact not only on the patient but also on close family members. Northouse and Swain (1987) examined the initial adjustment of patients and their husbands to the impact of the diagnosis of breast cancer. Future nursing research may continue to explore the diagnosis of cancer as a family crisis as well as an individual crisis.

Grieving. Grieving, according to Carpenito (1984), is a state in which an individual or family experiences an actual or a perceived loss of a person, object, function, status, or relationship; anticipatory grieving is the state in which an individual or family responds to the realization of a future loss. Grieving in cancer patients may be situational in that the grieving is related to the change in life style or to the knowledge that one has a terminal illness. In addition, there may be actual losses of body functions of body parts as a result of surgical treatment for cancer.

Nursing research about grieving follows two avenues. The first is about the grieving process and nursing interventions designed to promote bereavement resolution, and the second vein of research is concerned with oncology nurses who are constantly exposed to many terminal patients. The questions pursued in this latter line of research follow from concerns about nursing education and counseling that will help nurses better provide care for terminal patients or for patients who are experiencing a loss of a body part or function. Two studies that reflect these two avenues of research are summarized in the appendix (Padilla, Baker, & Dolan, 1977; Saunders, 1981).

Coping: Ineffective Individual. The nursing diagnosis of ineffective individual coping is defined as the state in which the individual experiences, or is at risk of experiencing, an inability to manage internal or environmental stressors adequately because of inadequate physical, psychological, or behavioral resources (Carpenito, 1983, 1984). This period of crisis may evolve into a set of potentially chronic stressful situations and decisions that relate to treatment and life style changes.

Singer (1984) states that the study of coping is governed by the way the researcher conceptualizes stress. According to Singer, the two major views of stress are the classic formulation, associated with the work of Selye (1956), identifying physiological and endocrinologic processes; and the interactionist view propounded by the work of Lazarus (Lazarus, 1966; Lazarus & Folkman, 1984) that includes physiological changes, but also includes an appraisal process with behavioral, cognitive, and emotional components. The key difference in these two views of stress, argues Singer, is in the location of the stressor. According to the Selye view, the stressor is outside the person; whereas the stressor is a mental construct according to the Lazarus view. In combining these two views, Singer advocates a three-part view of stress from the stressor through the transmission channels to the organism. Successful coping processes will generally reduce the stress, but in different ways depending on what is to be accomplished. Singer concludes that coping is usually regarded as a psychosocial adjustment to a stress. Where the stressor is health-related, the assessment of the effect of coping on physiological as well as psychosocial outcomes is relevant.

There are three basic assumptions of Lazarus' theory of coping (Lazarus & Folkman, 1984). They are as follows: (1) each person has a unique perception of any situation; (2) the perception of the situation interacts with the situation and with the individual's response to it; and (3) the evaluation of the situation is influenced by factors from within the individual and from the situation itself. The evaluation process is the element of appraisal. Interventions to promote coping may be derived from altering the situations or altering the appraisal of situations. Saunders and McCorkle (1987), using the framework on coping developed by Lazarus and Folkman, studied the coping responses and the use of social support by patients with newly diagnosed lung cancer. According to Saunders and McCorkle, patients use intrapsychic coping modes (altering the appraisal) as well as accepting medical treatment for coping with the diagnosis of lung cancer.

Studies of coping processes follow two general strategies according to Singer (1984). One type evolves from a theoretical position describing categories of possible coping behaviors. Instruments to measure coping behaviors are developed and studies compare the relative success of people using one type of coping behavior in contrast to using other coping behaviors. Cohen and Lazarus (1973, 1979) identify active coping processes that patients employ to cope with the stress of illness.

The second general strategy for studying coping processes, according to Singer, examines a given stress or stressor, such as cancer. Individuals who cope successfully are then contrasted for different behavioral patterns with those who do not, thereby leading to inferences about which behaviors are functionally more adaptive.

The work of Johnson (Johnson & Leventhal, 1974; Johnson, Christman, & Stitt, 1985) is concerned with interventions to promote coping by providing accurate information and expectations about stressful medical examinations and treatments. Johnson proposes that accurate information gives patients a measure of control over stressful situations. Janis (1983) also is interested in interventions to promote coping. His work describes the value of social support and anticipatory guidance as a method of promoting stress reduction. Thus we see research on coping and stress reduction may examine individual differences in coping as well as nursing intervention techniques to promote coping and health-care outcomes as dependent variables.

Knowledge Deficit: Disease and Treatments.   Patient teaching is an important component of nursing care of the cancer patient (Lauer, Murphy, & Powers, 1982). Nursing research about this problem may focus on aspects of information delivery, teaching methods, or content. The concept of "uncertainty" developed by Mischel (1983, 1984) also relates to understanding the nursing diagnosis of knowledge deficit.

Johnson has developed a line of nursing research involving the use of information about anticipated experiences to promote coping and recovery following noxious medical examinations or surgery (Johnson & Leventhal, 1974; Johnson, Christman, & Stitt, 1985). Johnson's intervention techniques consist of providing patients with certain types of information for reducing uncertainty and for creating a set of cognitively accurate expectations. By providing patients with appropriate information about what to expect, the nurse gives patients a measure of control over potentially unpleasant experiences. The providing of information as a nursing intervention reduces knowledge deficit experienced by patients and facilitates positive coping behavior. Johnson's line of nursing research has been highly influential on studies directed toward providing patients with appropriate information about their diseases and their treatments.

Two interesting studies related to knowledge deficits in cancer patients are summarized in the appendix. The article by Lauer, Murphy, & Powers (1982) is a study comparing nurses' perceptions of the knowledge patients have and need versus patients' actual knowledge and perceptions. This study is of interest because it highlights areas about which nurses may assume patients already have information when, in fact, they do not. The study also highlights areas about which nurses erroneously believe that patients lack information. The study by Dodd (1984a) deals with the impact of information about chemotherapy upon self-care behavior and actual knowledge. Knowledge and self-care behavior are dependent variables, varying according to the different types and amounts of information that is provided. In the Dodd study, nurses examine the impact that health teaching has upon subsequent patient behavior. Interventions to reduce knowledge deficits all appear to provide the patients with a sense of control over uncertainty.

Alteration in Nutrition: Less than Body Requirements. The nursing diagnosis of alteration in nutrition is defined as the state in which an individual experiences, or is at risk of experiencing, reduced weight related to inadequate intake of nutrients (Carpenito, 1983, 1984). Several etiologic or contributing factors qualify this nursing diagnosis. They are alteration in nutrition, less than body requirements caused by: anorexia; nausea and vomiting; or secondary to the disease process and treatments.

The American Cancer Society (1981), Burns (1982), and Grant (1984, 1987) have identified anorexia as a significant nursing care problem for oncology patients. This loss of appetite may be related to the disease process itself or to the chemotherapy or radiation therapy prescribed as treatment for the disease. The anorexia may also be symptomatic of underlying grief and depression. Nursing care research may center on the causes of the anorexia or on interventions designed to overcome anorexia in cancer patients (Dixon, 1984).

Grant (1987) has developed a theoretical framework to conceptualize anorexia during cancer and cancer treatment. The model defines physiological, psychological, and sociocultural determinants of anorexia. In Grant's framework anorexia is viewed as a decrease in appetite and a decrease in the ability to eat, both of which lead to a decrease in ingestion of food. Building upon her conceptual model, Grant developed a structured teaching program for intervention with head and neck oncology patients undergoing radiation therapy. An important theoretical finding resulting from Grant's research is that both a subjective measure of appetite and an objective measure of dietary intake are necessary for accurate descriptions of anorexia in oncology patients.

As with anorexia, nausea and vomiting are identified as significant nursing care problems for the oncology patient, both because of the discomfort these symptoms cause and also because of the potential adverse impact on nutrition resulting from nausea and vomiting (American Cancer Society, 1981; Burns, 1982; Burish & Redd, 1983; Zeltzer & LeBaron, 1983).

Nurses may become involved in collaborative research to explore what interventions may overcome nausea and vomiting in the cancer patient undergoing treatment. One such example of a collaborative research venture is the study summarized in the appendix (Bishop et al, 1984). In this study, a randomized, double-blind format was used to administer an antiemetic drug in patients undergoing cancer chemotherapy. Patients who received an active antiemetic drug experienced less actual nausea and vomiting and also reported experiencing less anxiety while receiving the active antiemetic drug in contrast to a placebo.

Unfortunately, no antiemetic drugs have been found to be completely effective and free of undesirable side effects for all patients undergoing chemotherapy treatments for cancer (Cotanch & Strum, 1987). Cotanch and her colleagues have found that relaxation through self-hypnosis (Cotanch, Hockenberry, & Herman, 1985) and progressive muscle relaxation techniques (Cotanch & Strum, 1987) are successful behavioral intervention techniques for children receiving cancer chemotherapy. The theoretical framework employed by Cotanch emphasizes the patient's appraisal of the situation. By teaching patients to use relaxation techniques, Cotanch is providing the patients with a way to maintain some control over an otherwise stressful situation. Continuing research into behavioral interventions for nausea and vomiting in cancer chemotherapy appears to be a valuable direction for dealing with this problem.

Alterations in Comfort: Pain. Providing relief for the patient in pain is an important activity of the oncology nurse. Nursing research in relation to pain management often involves noninvasive techniques for pain relief (Anderson, 1982). Research using techniques that give patients a perception of control (Johnson, Christman, & Stitt, 1985) as described above in the research by Cotanch may also prove to be a useful theoretical framework for pain management.

Providing pain relief also involves collaborations among nurses giving nursing care. Some nurses are more knowledgeable than others about behavioral intervention techniques to control pain. Research into nurses' decision making in the administration of pain medications may highlight the need for appropriate nursing assessment of pain and the appropriate use of both behavioral and physiological pain control techniques by nurses.

Understanding of the physiological mechanisms involved in the pain process is important for nurses who are exercising discretion over the use of various pain control techniques. A current conceptualization of the pain process is known as the "gate control theory of pain" (Melzack & Wall, 1965; Donovan, 1982). The gate control theory states that the experience of pain results from the combined action of both neurotransmitters and neuromodulators at each neuroreceptor site from the source of injury to the cortex. Nursing research on noninvasive techniques for moderating cancer pain may combine behavioral and physiological theoretical frameworks by devising interventions that somehow interrupt the action of the neurotransmitters and neuromodulators (Donovan, 1982; Feldman, 1984).

Self-Concept: Disturbance in Body Image. Nursing research on changes in body image has relevance for the study of treatments for cancer. Specifically, surgical treatment for cancer often is debilitating at best and perhaps results in the loss of a vital body part or function, as with amputation or colostomy (Follick, Smith & Turk, 1984). Moreover, treatment with chemotherapy may result in total body hair loss for prolonged periods of time. Also, permanent indwelling catheters (eg, Broviac or Hickman) are being used with increasing frequency for chemotherapy patients, especially children. All of these treatment modalities may result in disturbances of the body image for oncology patients.

The goal of cancer nursing research about disturbances in body image is to develop useful intervention strategies to facilitate the acceptance of altered body images or altered body functions. However, nursing research is also necessary to define and describe the variety of patient responses in order to develop appropriate interventions. For example, Meyerowitz (1983) studied the responses of women who had been treated surgically for breast cancer during the preceding 3½ years. She found that the level of cancer-specific denial emerged as the variable most strongly associated with distress following the mastectomy. A series of studies that reveal a great deal of data about the responses of cancer patients treated with a colostomy are the reports of the Quality Assurance Program for Cancer Nursing (QAPCN) research project (Padilla, 1985).

Changes in body image are not confined to cancer patients only. Such changes are a normal part of growth and development, particularly for adolescents. However, for teen-agers with cancer, the changes and the threats to self-esteem that accompany treatment for cancer may be profound. Therefore a worthy area for future nursing research would be to use theories of adolescent development for examining the responses of teen-agers to body image changes associated with treatment for cancer.

Powerlessness Related to Inability to Control Situations. The nursing diagnosis of powerlessness is defined as the state in which an individual perceives a lack of personal control over certain events or situations (Carpenito, 1983,

1984). Oncology patients may experience powerlessness either as a result of the situation in which they find themselves (eg, hospitalization), or a result of pathophysiologic processes that may be progressively debilitating and possibly terminal.

Studies of loss of personal control during hospitalization may examine individual differences in the desire for control over procedures and treatments. Smith et al (1984) have studied this concept.

Research may also focus on patient satisfaction as an important issue related to powerlessness. Two studies summarized in the appendix relate to patient satisfaction. One article is by La Monica, et al (1986). This article describes three studies to develop a patient satisfaction instrument. A second approach to patient satisfaction is summarized in the appendix (Lauer, Murphy, & Powers, 1982); this matches the learning needs of cancer patients with the perceptions of learning needs by nursing staff. The argument could be made that patient satisfaction within a hospital experience may vary inversely with perceived powerlessness within the situation.

As with body image changes, issues of personal control are particularly prominent during the years of adolescence. The coping methods used by teen-age oncology patients to overcome feelings of powerlessness within the hospital setting constitute a potentially valuable area for oncology nursing research. Related to coping with powerlessness is the concept of change. Haase (1987) has conducted a qualitative study to develop the theoretical concept of courage among chronically ill adolescents. Included in her sample are teen-age oncology patients. Haase has found that a sense of growth, creativity, and mastery are the resolution of the phenomenon of courage expressed by chronically ill adolescents.

One way of studying the nursing diagnosis of powerlessness is to follow the theoretical formulation known as "learned helplessness." This concept was originally developed in the work of Seligman (1975) and extended theoretically in the statement by Abramson, Seligman, and Teasdale (1978). The theoretical premise of learned helplessness is that when one is exposed continually to unpredictable and unavoidable adverse experiences, the results are behaviors that appear to be depression. Much social science research has substantiated the observations and predictions of the concept of learned helplessness. The study by Lewis (1982) summarized in the appendix contains an innovative example of applying the model of learned helplessness to the study of quality of life in late-stage cancer patients.

Social Support

Social support is a concept related to the adjustment of cancer patients to the long-term effects of their disease. Relevant nursing diagnoses that cluster about the concept of social support include social isolation caused by cancer; social interactions, impaired; and alterations of family functioning (Carpenito, 1984).

Social support includes professional and informal networks, including the patient's family and community connections. Social support is not a unitary concept but is multidimensional (Suls, 1982; and DiMatteo & Hays, 1981). Nevertheless, several studies point to the fact that social support is an important variable that influences patient adherence to medical regimens and successful coping with a medical problem (Caplan et al, 1979; Janis, 1983; Saltzer, 1980; Suls, 1982; Wallston et al, 1983; Wortman, 1984).

A thorough review of the concept of social support as it applies specifically to coping with cancer is provided by Wortman (1984). According to Wortman, regardless of the strengths and weaknesses of individual studies, findings in the literature are consistent in concluding that social support may be a significant resource for coping with cancer. One of the ironies of the problems experienced by patients with cancer is that at a time when patients experience the greatest anxieties and fears about it, they may also have great interpersonal difficulties that interfere with obtaining adequate social support (Wortman, 1984).

Tilden (1985) also reviews the issues related to the study of social support but specifically tailors her review to the use of this concept for nursing theory. Basically, Tilden identifies the same issues as Wortman, but in addition she considers theory development as a link to future nursing practice. Familiarity with these general issues is important for the researcher planning to use the concept of social support as part of a theoretical framework for cancer nursing research.

Nurses, and researchers from related social science disciplines, have grappled with the conceptual and methodological issues related to social support. Weinert, a nurse, has developed a social support measure called the PRQ85 (Weinert, 1987). The letters PRQ stand for Personal Resource Questionnaire. The PRQ85 is the latest version of Weinert's scale. Future cancer nursing research testing the PRQ85 with oncology patients would provide useful information about the scale as well as about the concept of social support.

Dunkel–Schetter, Wortman, and Olviedo (1984) defined social support as having three components: the provision of (1) useful information and advice; (2) assistance with tasks; and (3) emotional sustenance to another individual. For the cancer patient, social support may be provided by family, friends, physicians, and nurses. In studying patients with either breast cancer or colorectal cancer, Dunkel–Schetter, Wortman, and Olviedo found that most patients received adequate social support; but for about one quarter of the population studied, significant interpersonal difficulties were associated with the disease. The patients most likely to have difficulties in the area of social support were those with more advanced disease and poorer physical condition.

Rawnsley (1982) has proposed a theoretical nursing model for brief psychotherapy for persons with recurrent cancer. Rawnsley's view of the need for brief psychotherapy is really a theoretical framework for the purposes of social support in the care of cancer patients. Nursing research is needed to test and evaluate Rawnsley's model as well as to evaluate the positive effects of cancer self-help groups upon selected patient variables, such as adherence to medical regimens, emotional state, quality of life, and longevity.

Adherence to Prescribed Regimens

Several relevant nursing diagnoses for treatment of the cancer patient relate to adherence to prescribed regimens. These diagnoses are alterations in health maintenance; self-care deficits; and finally, knowledge deficits (Carpenito, 1984). Several models discussed in the earlier section on primary prevention are also useful for studying compliance with treatments, an aspect of secondary prevention in cancer patients. It is important to recognize that cancer may be viewed as a chronic illness with cycles of acute and controlled phases. These cycles of illness and remission may be due either to the disease process itself or to the consequences of medical oncology therapy. The issues of adherence to prescribed regimens are important for understanding secondary prevention, but the models also apply to tertiary prevention (rehabilitation) as well.

Locus of Control. Described in depth earlier in the chapter, studies of locus of control from the perspective of primary prevention generally measure the main outcome as acquisition of health knowledge and also adherence to healthy life styles or healthy regimens. When considering locus of control in secondary prevention, the dependent variable frequently is adherence to a long-term prescribed medical regimen.

In viewing cancer as a chronic disease we can find examples of studies about other chronic illnesses and prescribed medical regimens in which locus of control is the principle variable in determining the outcome. Witenberg et al (1983) have studied perceptions of control and causality as a prediction of compliance with dialysis. They have found that perceived control is associated with positive coping but is unrelated to compliance.

Saltzer (1981) studied compliance of obese female patients with a prescribed medical weight loss regimen. Internals who highly valued physical appearance were the most likely to succeed at their initial weight loss goals. In addition, Saltzer's Weight Locus of Control (WLOC) scale (1982b) has been used to predict behaviors directed toward maintenance of weight among oncology patients undergoing treatment (Grant, 1987).

Shillinger (1983) describes implications for clinical nursing practice by relating internal locus of control to self-care and suggests that individuals with external locus of control expectancies may fall into the nursing diagnostic category of self-care deficit. Clearly, future research for cancer nursing may fruitfully explore the theoretical concept of locus of control, an important variable for predicting adherence behaviors for the chronically ill.

Predicting Adherence Behavior: Other Models. Several other theoretical models that were discussed in the section on primary prevention are also useful for studying secondary prevention and cancer patient care. Taylor, Lichtman, and Wood (1984) studied compliance with chemotherapy among patients with breast cancer. They found a high rate of compliance (92 percent) because of the perceived centrality of the treatment to recovery.

Nevertheless, predicting individual differences in adherence is an important area of research. Padilla and Grant (1983) used the Health Belief Model, described earlier, to predict the adherence behavior of cancer patients treatment.

Saltzer (1981, 1982a) used the theory of reasoned action (Fishbein & Ajzen, 1975) to study adherence to a prescribed medical regimen for weight reduction.

This theory may prove useful for studying the adherence behaviors of cancer patients as well.

The study by Dodd (1984a) summarized in the appendix describes a randomized experimental study designed to measure the content and type of information used by chemotherapy patients to promote knowledge of chemotherapy and self-care behavior. This study combines theoretical frameworks from self-care concepts (Orem, 1980) as well as building upon the work in stress reduction by Johnson and Leventhal (1974). In addition, Dodd's study includes the concept that information is an aspect of situational control as proposed by Rotter (1966) in relation to the construct of locus of control.

TERTIARY PREVENTION: REHABILITATION

Tertiary prevention, as defined earlier, refers to the rehabilitation or adjustment after treatment for disease. As survival rates improve, cancer patients more frequently resemble chronically ill rather than acutely ill patients (Aiken, 1976; Burns, 1982; Driever, 1982; Georgiadou, 1982; Germino, 1982; Mages & Mendelsohn, 1979; McCorkle & Benoliel, 1981; and McLaughlin, 1982). Thus, rehabilitation from cancer is becoming an increasingly significant area of research.

Several interrelated topics are of major concern for the nurse whose research principally focuses upon tertiary prevention. These main categories of interest are quality of life, social support, and survival.

Quality of Life

Quality of life is an important outcome variable of cancer treatment and rehabilitation. In most studies conceptual frameworks for quality of life emphasize two aspects: objective outcomes, such as functional deficits, and subjective outcomes, such as satisfaction with perceived quality of life. Early measures of quality of life tended to focus on performance as exemplified by the Karnofsky performance status (Karnofsky & Burchenal, 1949), a classic reference. Today, however, the idea of quality of life in cancer patients is expanded to be a composite variable of all elements of life styles for the cancer patient (Grieco & Long, 1984).

Meyerowitz (1983) examined post-mastectomy coping strategies and related these strategies to outcome measures signifying quality of life. The Lewis study (1982) that is summarized in the appendix examined quality of life in late-stage cancer patients.

A cluster of nursing studies examine cancer patient responses to psychosocial variables (Driever, 1982; Georgiadou, 1982; and McCorkle & Benoliel, 1981). These studies compare cancer patients with heart disease patients on a variety of psychosocial variables and follow their principal patient concerns over an extended period of time from 3 months to 6 months.

Padilla, et al (1983) developed a quality-of-life index for cancer patients. This index was used in the nursing research project known as the Quality

Assurance Program for Cancer Nursing (Padilla, 1985), which examined quality of life as one of the major outcome variables for cancer patients who received a colostomy as part of their treatment.

Social Support

Closely related to the issue of quality of life in adjustment to cancer is the concept of social support. Nurses have been pioneers in the form of social support that has become the hospice movement for care of patients with terminal cancer. The underlying theme for the hospice movement is "death with dignity." Terminal patients may actually reside in a physical setting known as a hospice or they may be cared for at home by close family members or friends who receive social support for their efforts from members of a hospice program. Future nursing research should endeavor to evaluate both qualitatively and quantitatively the perceived quality of life as experienced by patients and their families who participate in hospice care versus hospital care for terminal oncology patients.

Nurses have also been closely involved with the promotion of self-care groups such as colostomy clubs or mastectomy clubs. Nursing interventions for the nursing diagnosis of "knowledge deficit of support agencies and self-care programs" (Carpenito, 1983, 1984) include the referral of identified patients to these groups as part of rehabilitation. The concept of social support, as described earlier in the section on secondary prevention, is a potential theoretical framework for research evaluating the success of these programs.

Survival

Fortunately, the diagnosis of cancer is no longer an automatic terminal diagnosis. A great number of cancer patients live in a disease-free state for years after treatment. Many of these long-term survivors are actually considered to be cured of cancer. As the length of survival and the number of survivors of cancer continue to increase, research is needed to identify the main issues related to this dimension. At present, research on survival is a small but growing area of interest for oncology nursing research.

In the area of childhood cancer, the growth in the number of survivors has been dramatic in recent years (Klopovich, 1983; Ruccione & Fergusson, 1984). According to Klopovich (1983), the constantly improving prognosis for children with cancer has altered the focus of care to assisting the patient to live with chronic illness. Klopovich has identified four important areas of research about survivors of childhood cancer. They are school reentry, nonmedical costs of illness, marital stress and divorce among parents of childhood cancer patients, and long-term compliance with treatment.

Nurses have the potential to influence patient expectancies about survival by their behavior toward cancer patients. Whelan (1984) examined the attitudes of oncology nurses in England and the United States toward cancer treatment and survival. She found oncology nurses held pessimistic views about the diagnosis of cancer in general, but that the attitudes toward specific types of cancer vary according to the site of the disease. Whelan recommends that oncology nurses receive inservice education that provides more information about the success of various types of cancer treatments along with actual contact with patients who have been successfully treated and cured of their disease.

Although nursing research about survival of cancer is still very much at the descriptive stage, Stoner and Keampfer (1985) have used the concept of hope as a theoretical framework related to recalled life expectancy for the study of oncology patients. They used a scale to measure hope known as the Stoner Hope Scale (Stoner, 1982). The findings of Stoner and Keampfer have implications for the communication of life-expectancy information to patients.

Nurses may draw upon theoretical frameworks developed for the care of patients with other diseases for the successful study of survival by cancer patients. One possible framework is the concept of "redesigning the dream" that was developed by Mischel and Murdaugh (1987) for explaining the process of family adjustment to heart transplantation. This process has three phases, immersion, passage, and negotiation. The phase of negotiation corresponds to the stage of recovery and may prove to be relevant for understanding the adjustments that cancer patients and their families make after surviving the acute treatment stage of illness.

The study of survival is an important new area for oncology nursing research. This research is related to the changing view of cancer from a terminal disease to a chronic disease. Issues relevant to survival of cancer are important to be studied in adults as well as children. We are indeed fortunate to be practicing in a time when the survival of cancer is a focus for research. Enhancing survival is the ultimate promise of oncology research.

SUMMARY AND CONCLUSION

In conclusion, this chapter has focused upon examples of theoretical frameworks used to study cancer patients in nursing research. As a way of organizing the chapter, the theories are categorized according to whether their principal usage is for studying primary prevention, secondary prevention, or tertiary prevention. These divisions in the chapter are strictly an organizational scheme. Certainly, each of the theoretical frameworks described may be creatively applied to any aspect of oncology nursing research.

When one is endeavoring to determine how a theoretical framework is used in a given research report, it is important to examine the review of the literature portion of the article, for in this section, the main theories that guide the research are identified and organized in relation to one another. The review of the literature weaves together the ideas that have influenced the author and sets the context for the specific research questions to be asked.

Remember, any single research project may use or combine several theories to create the specific theoretical framework for the research questions to be examined. Two of the studies summarized in the Appendix provide excellent examples of the value of tying together several theoretical ideas in the specific framework. The studies by Dodd (1984a) and by Lewis (1982) demonstrate the mechanisms of combining multiple ideas into theoretical frameworks that result in specific hypotheses.

The theoretical framework also governs the analysis of the results of research. This is especially important for qualitative research. An example in the Appendix of a qualitative study that leads to the generation of a new theoretical concept is the study by Saunders (1981), which develops the concept of "uncoupled identity" for bereavement resolution.

Whether one is using a quantitative or a qualitative methodology for research, it is important to relate the results and the conclusions to the original theoretical framework. Researchers should consider how the findings validate or refute theory at the conclusion of a research study to enhance the generalizability of the results.

As a final reminder, the most important effort that a researcher can make when developing a study is to "immerse" her- or himself in the theories relevant to the topic to be examined. Understanding how others have viewed and studied a topic allows a researcher to build upon work that has already been completed. Knowledge of relevant theories helps identify both the conceptual and methodological issues that surround a problem to be studied. A thorough comprehension of applicable theories is essential for successful research.

REFERENCES

Abramson, L.Y., Seligman, M.E.P., Teasdale, J.D. (1978). Learned helplessness in humans: Critique and reformulation. *Journal of Abnormal Psychology, 87*, 49–74.

Aiken, L.H. (1976). Chronic illness and responsive ambulatory care. In D. Mechanic (Ed.), *The growth of bureaucratic medicine.* New York: Wiley.

Ajzen, I., & Fishbein, M. (1980). *Understanding attitudes and predicting social behavior.* Englewood Cliffs, NJ: Prentice-Hall.

Alagna, S.W., & Reddy, D.M. (1984). Predictors of proficient technique and successful lesion detection in breast self-examination. *Health Psychology, 3*, 113–127.

American Cancer Society. (1981). *A cancer source book for nurses* (Rev. ed.). New York: American Cancer Society.

Anderson, B.L., Karlsson, J.A., Anderson, B., et al (1984). Anxiety and cancer treatment: Response to stressful radiotherapy. *Health Psychology, 3*, 535–551.

Anderson, J.L. (1982). Nursing management of the cancer patient in pain: A review of the literature. *Cancer Nursing, 5*(1), 33–41.

Anisman, H., & Zacharko, R.M. (1983). Stress and neoplasia: Speculations and caveats. *Behavioral Medicine Update, 5*, 27–35.

Artinian, B.M. (1982). Conceptual mapping: Development of the strategy. *Western Journal of Nursing Research, 4*, 379–393.

Atkinson, J.W. (1964). *An introduction to motivation.* Princeton: Van Nostrand.

Auger, J.R. (1976). *Behavioral systems and nursing.* Englewood Cliffs, NJ: Prentice-Hall.

Bandura, A. (1977). Self-efficacy: Toward a unifying theory of behavioral change. *Psychological Review, 84*, 191–215.

Becker, M.H., & Maiman, L.A. (1975). Sociobehavioral determinants of compliance with health and medical care recommendations. *Medical Care, 13*, 10–24.

Becker, M.N., Maiman, L.A., Kirscht, J.P., et al (1977). The health belief model and prediction of dietary compliance: A field experiment. *Journal of Health and Social Behavior, 18*, 348–366.

Bieliauskas, L.A. (1983). Considerations of depression and stress in the etiology of cancer. *Behavioral Medicine Update, 5*, 23–26.

Bishop, J.F., Olver, I.N., Wolf, M.M., et al (1984). Lorazepam: A randomized, double-blind, crossover study of a new antiemetic in patients receiving cytotoxic chemotherapy and prochlorperazine. *Journal of Clinical Oncology, 2*, 691–695.

Burish, T.G., & Redd, W.H. (1983). Behavioral approaches to reducing conditioned responses to chemotherapy in adult cancer patients. *Behavioral Medicine Update, 5*, 12–16.

Burns, N. (1982). *Nursing and cancer*. Philadelphia: Saunders.

Campbell, C. (1984). *Nursing diagnosis and intervention in nursing practice* (2nd ed.). New York: Wiley.

Caplan, R.D., Robinson, E.A.R., French, J.R.P., Jr., et al (1979). *Adhering to medical regimens: Pilot experiments in patient education and social support*. Ann Arbor, MI: Institute for Social Research.

Carpenito, L.J. (1983). *Nursing diagnosis: Application to clinical practice*. Philadelphia: Lippincott.

Carpenito, L.J. (1984). *Handbook of nursing diagnosis*. Philadelphia: Lippincott.

Cohen, F., & Lazarus, R.S. (1973). Active coping processes, coping dispositions, and recovery from surgery. *Psychosomatic Medicine, 35*, 375–389.

Cohen, F., & Lazarus, R. (1979). Coping with the stress of illness. In G.S. Stone, F. Cohen, N.E. Adler (Eds.), *Health psychology—A handbook* (217–254). San Francisco: Jossey-Bass.

Condiotte, M.M., & Lichtenstein. (1981) Self-efficacy and relapse in smoking cessation programs. *Journal of Consulting and Clinical Psychology, 49*, 648–658.

Conway, T.L., Vickers, R.R., Jr., Ward, H.W., et al (1981). Occupational stress and variation in cigarette, coffee, and alcohol consumption. *Journal of Health and Social Behavior, 22*, 155–165.

Cotanch, P., Hockenberry, M., Herman, S. (1985). Self-hypnosis as antiemetic therapy in children receiving chemotherapy. *Oncology Nursing Forum, 12*(4), 41–46.

Cotanch, P.H., & Sturm, S. (1987). Progressive muscle relaxation as antiemetic therapy for cancer patients. *Oncology Nursing Forum, 14*(1), 33–37.

Derdiarian, A.K. (1983). An instrument for theory and research development using the behavioral systems model for nursing: The cancer patient, (Part I). *Nursing Research, 32*, 196–201.

Derdiarian, A.K., & Forsythe, A.B. (1983). An instrument for theory and research development using the behavioral systems model for nursing: The cancer patient, (Part II). *Nursing Research, 32*, 260–266.

DiMatteo, M.R., & Hays, R. (1981). Social support and serious illness. In B.H. Gottlieb (Ed.), *Social networks and social support* (117–148). Beverly Hills: Sage.

Dixon, J. (1984). Effect of nursing interventions on nutritional and performance status in cancer patients. *Nursing Research, 33*, 330–335.

Dodd, M.J. (1984a). Measuring informational intervention for chemotherapy knowledge and self-care behavior. *Research in Nursing and Health, 7*, 43–50.

Dodd, M.J. (1984b). Patterns of self-care in cancer patients receiving radiation therapy. *Oncology Nursing Forum, 11*(3), 23–27.

Dohrenwend, B.S., & Dohrenwend, B.P. (Eds.). (1974). Stressful life events: Their nature and effects. New York: Wiley.

Donovan, M. (1982). Cancer pain: You can help. *Nursing Clinics of North America, 17,* 713–728.

Driever, M.J. (1982). Patient concerns at three and six months post diagnosis. In MV Batey (Ed.), *Communicating nursing research: Proceedings of the western society for research in nursing conference, 15,* 140–141.

Dunkel-Schetter, C., Wortman, C.B., Olviedo, M. (1984). Social support and adjustment to cancer. *Cancer Focus, 7*(4), 58–60.

Fawcett, J. (1984). *Analysis and evaluation of conceptual models of nursing.* Philadelphia: Davis.

Feldman, H.R. (1984). Psychological differentiation and the phenomenon of pain. *Advances in Nursing Science, 6,* 50–57.

Fishbein, M., & Ajzen, I. (1975). *Belief, attitude, intention and behavior: An introduction to theory and research.* Reading, MA: Addison-Wesley.

Follick, M.J., Smith, T.W., Turk, D.C. (1984). Psychosocial adjustment following ostomy. *Health Psychology, 3,* 505–517.

Frank-Stromborg, M., Wright, P.S., Segalla, M., et al (1984). Psychological impact of the "cancer" diagnosis. *Oncology Nursing Forum, 11*(3), 16–22.

Georgiadou, F. (1982). Enforced social dependency and life threatening events. In MV Batey (Ed.), *Communicating nursing research: Proceedings of the western society for research in nursing.* Boulder, Colorado: Western Interstate Commission for Higher Education, *15,* 138–139.

Germino, B.B. (1982). Acknowledged awareness of life threatening illness. In MV Batey (Ed.), *Communicating nursing research: Proceedings of the western society for research in nursing conference, 15,* 137–138.

Glaser, B.G., & Strauss, A.L. (1967). *The discovery of grounded theory: Strategies for qualitative research.* New York: Aldine.

Grant, M. (1984). *Anorexia in head and neck cancer patients undergoing radiation therapy.* Unpublished manuscript.

Grant, M.M. (1987). *Effects of a structured teaching program for cancer patients undergoing head and neck radiation therapy on anorexia, nutritional status, functional status, treatment response, and quality of life.* Unpublished doctoral dissertation, University of California, San Francisco.

Green, L.W. (1970). Should health education abandon attitude change strategies? Perspective from recent research. *Health Education Monographs, 30,* 25–47.

Grieco, A., & Long, C.J. (1984). Investigation of the Karnofsky performance status as a measure of quality of life. *Health Psychology, 3,* 129–142.

Haase, J.E. (1987). Components of courage in chronically ill adolescents: A phenomenological study. *Advances in Nursing Science, 9*(2), 64–80.

Heider, F. (1958). *The psychology of interpersonal relations.* New York: Wiley.

Holland, W., & Karhausen, L. (1979). Health care and epidemiology. London: Kimpton Medical Publications.

Holmes, T.H., & Rahe, R.H. (1967). The social readjustment rating scale. *Journal of Psychosomatic Research, 11,* 213–218.

Horan, M.L. (1982). Parental reaction to the birth of an infant with a defect: An attributional approach. *Advances in Nursing Science, 5,* 57–68.

Janis, I.L. (1983). The role of social support in adherence to stressful decisions. *American Psychologist, 38,* 143–160.

Janz, N., & Becker, M. (1984). A health belief model: A decade later. *Health Education Quarterly, 11*(1), 1–47.

Johnson, D.E. (1959). The nature of a science of nursing. *Nursing Outlook, 7,* 291–294.

Johnson, J.E., Christman, N.J., Stitt, C. (1985). Personal control interventions: Short and long-term effects on surgical patients. *Research in Nursing and Health, 8,* 131–145.

Johnson, J., & Leventhal, H. (1974). Effects of accurate expectations and behavioral instructions on reactions during a noxious medical examination. *Journal of Personality and Social Psychology, 29,* 710–718.

Jones, E.E., & Davis, K.E. (1965). From acts to dispositions: The attribution process in person perception. In L. Berkowitz (Ed.), *Advances in experimental social psychology* (Vol. 2, 219–266). New York: Academic Press.

Karnofsky, D.A., & Burchenal, J.H. (1949). The clinical evaluation of chemotherapeutic agents in cancer. In C.M. MacLeod (Ed.), *Evaluation of chemotherapeutic agents.* New York: Columbia Press.

Kegeles, S.S. (1983). Behavioral methods for effective cancer screening and prevention. *Behavioral Medicine Update, 5,* 36–44.

Kelley, H.H. (1967). Attribution theory in social psychology. In D. Levine (Ed.), *Nebraska symposium on motivation, 1967.* Lincoln: University of Nebraska Press.

Kim, M.J., McFarland, G.K., McLane, A.M. (1984). *Pocket guide to nursing diagnoses.* St. Louis; Mosby.

Klagsbrun, S.C. (1970). Cancer, emotion, and nurses. *American Journal of Psychiatry, 126,* 1237–1244.

Klopovich, P.M. (1983). Research on problems of chronicity in childhood cancer. *Oncology Nursing Forum, 10*(3), 72–75.

Kobasa, S.C. (1982). The hardy personality: Toward a social psychology of stress and health. In G.S. Sanders & J. Suls (Eds.), *Social psychology of health and illness* (3–32). Hillsdale, NJ: Lawrence Erlbaum.

LaMonica, E.L., Oberst, M.T., Madea, A.R., et al (1986). Development of a patient satisfaction scale. *Research in Nursing and Health, 9,* 43–50.

Lauer, P., Murphy, S.P., Powers, M.J. (1982). Learning needs of cancer patients: A comparison of nurse and patient perceptions. *Nursing Research, 31,* 11–16.

Lazarus, R.S. (1966). *Psychological stress and the coping process.* New York: McGraw-Hill.

Lazarus, R., & Folkman, S. (1984). *Stress, appraisal, and coping.* New York: Springer.

Lefcourt, H.M. (Ed.). (1981). *Research with the locus of control construct. Vol. 1. Assessment methods.* New York: Academic Press.

Lefcourt, H.M. (1982). *Locus of control: Current trends in theory and research* (2nd ed.). Hillsdale, NJ: Lawrence Erlbaum.

Levenson, H. (1973). Multidimensional locus of control in psychiatric patients. *Journal of Consulting and Clinical Psychology, 41,* 397–404.

Levenson, H. (1974). Activism and powerful others: Distinctions within the concept of internal–external control. *Journal of Personality Assessment, 38,* 377–383.

Leventhal, H. (1970). Findings and theory in the study of fear communications. In L. Berkowitz (Ed.), *Advances in experimental social psychology* (Vol. 5). New York: Academic Press.

Leventhal, H., Safer, M.A., Panagis, D.M. (1983). The impact of communications on the self-regulations of health beliefs, decisions, and behavior. *Health Education Quarterly, 10*(1), 3–29.

Lewis, F.M. (1982). Experienced personal control and quality of life in late-stage cancer patients. *Nursing Research, 31,* 113–119.

Mages, N.L., & Mendelsohn, G.A. (1979). Effects of cancer on patients' lives: A personological approach. In G.C. Stone, F. Cohen, N.F. Adler (Eds.), *Health Psychology* (255-284). San Francisco: Jossey-Bass.

Maiman, L.A., & Becker, M.H. (1974). The health belief model: Origin and correlates in psychological theory. *Health Education Monographs*, 336-353.

McCorkle, R., & Benoliel, J.Q. (1981). *Cancer patient responses to psychosocial variables.* Seattle: University of Washington, School of Nursing.

McIntyre, K.O., Lichtenstein, E., Mermelstein, R.J. (1983). Self-efficacy and relapse in smoking cessation: A replication and extension. *Journal of Consulting and Clinical Psychology, 51,* 632-633.

McLaughlin, J.S. (1982). Toward a theoretical model for community health programs. *Advances in Nursing Science, 5,* 7-28.

Mechanic, D. (1972). Social psychologic factors affecting the presentation of bodily complaints. *New England Journal of Medicine, 286,* 1132-1139.

Mechanic, D. (1975). Sociocultural and social-psychological factors affecting personal responses to psychological disorder. *Journal of Health and Social Behavior, 16,* 393-404.

Melzack, R., & Wall, P.D. (1965). Pain mechanisms: A new theory. *Science, 150,* 971-979.

Meyerowitz, B.E. (1983). Postmastectomy coping strategies and quality of life. *Health Psychology, 2,* 117-132.

Mischel, M.H. (1983). Adjusting the fit: Development of uncertainty scales for specific clinical populations. *Western Journal of Nursing Research, 5,* 355-370.

Mischel, M.H. (1984). Perceived uncertainty and stress in illness. *Research in Nursing and Health, 7,* 163-171.

Mischel, M.H., & Murdaugh, C.L. (1987). Family adjustment to heart transplantation: Redesigning the dream. *Nursing Research, 36,* 332-338.

Moos, R.H., & Tsu, V.D. (1977). The crisis of physical illness: An overview. In R.H. Moos (Ed.), *Coping with physical illness* (3-21). New York: Plenum Press.

Northouse, L.L., & Swain, M.A. (1987). Adjustment of patients and husbands to the initial impact of breast cancer. *Nursing Research, 36*(4), 221-225.

Orem, D.C. (1980). *Nursing: Concepts of practice* (2nd ed.). New York: McGraw-Hill.

Padilla, G.V. (1985). Final report of the Quality assurance program for cancer nursing grant, NU00849 for 1981-84. Bethesda, MD: Division of Nursing, United States Public Health Service.

Padilla, G.V., & Grant, M.M. (1983). Final report of Compliance strategies for cancer therapy grant, CA31164 for 1983-1986. Bethesda, MD: National Cancer Institute.

Padilla, G.V., Baker, V.E., Dolan, V. (1977). Interacting with dying patients. In M.V. Batey (Ed.), *Communicating nursing research: Proceedings of the western society for research in nursing conference, 8,* 101-114. Boulder, Colorado: Western Interstate Commission for Higher Education.

Padilla, G.V., Presant, C., Grant, M.M., et al (1983). Quality of life index for patients with cancer. *Research in Nursing and Health, 6,* 117-126.

Pennebaker, J.W. (1982). *The psychology of physical symptoms.* New York: Springer-Verlag.

Pennebaker, J.W., & Skelton, J.A. (1978). Psychological parameters of physical symptoms. *Personality and Social Psychology Bulletin, 4,* 524-530.

Phares, E.J. (1976). *Locus of control in personality.* Morristown, NJ: General Learning Press.

Rawnsley, M.M. (1982). Brief psychotherapy for persons with recurrent cancer: A holistic practice model. *Advances in Nursing Science, 5,* 69-76.

Riehl, J.P., & Roy, C. (1980). *Conceptual models for nursing practice* (2nd ed.). New York: Appleton-Century-Crofts.

Rodin, J. (1978). Somatopsychics and attribution. *Personality and Social Psychology Bulletin, 4*, 531-540.

Rosenstock, I.M. (1966). Why people use health services. *Milbank Memorial Fund Quarterly, 44*, 94-124.

Rosenstock, I.M. (1974). The Health Belief Model and preventive health behavior. *Health Education Monographs, 2*, 354-396.

Rosenstock, I.M., & Kirscht, J.P. (1974). Practice implications. *Health Education Monographs, 2*, 470-473.

Rotter, J.B. (1954). *Social learning and clinical psychology.* New Jersey: Prentice-Hall.

Rotter, J.B. (1966). Generalized expectancies for internal versus external control or reinforcement. *Psychological Monographs, 80*, (1, Whole No. 609).

Rotter, J.B. (1974). Some problems and misconceptions related to the construct of internal versus external control of reinforcement. *Journal of Consulting and Clinical Psychology, 43*, 56-57.

Ruccione, K., & Fergusson, J. (1984). Late effects of childhood cancer and its treatment. *Oncology Nursing Forum, 11*(5), 54-64.

Saltzer, E.B. (1980). Social determinants of successful weight loss: An analysis of behavioral intentions and actual behavior. *Basic and Applied Social Psychology, 1*, 329-342.

Saltzer, E.B. (1981). Cognitive moderations of the relationship between behavioral intentions and behavior. *Journal of Personality and Social Psychology, 41*, 260-271.

Saltzer, E.B. (1982a). The relationship of personal efficacy beliefs to behavior. *The British Journal of Social and Clinical Psychology, 21*, 213-221.

Saltzer, E.B. (1982b). The weight locus of control (WLOC) scale: A specific measure of locus of control with respect to weight. *Journal of Personality Assessment, 46*, 620-628.

Saltzer, E.B., & Saltzer, E.I. (1987). Internal control and health. *Western Journal of Nursing Research, 9*, 542-554.

Saunders, J.M. (1981). A process of bereavement resolution: Uncoupled identity. *Western Journal of Nursing Research, 3*, 321-331.

Saunders, J.M., & McCorkle, R. (1987). Social support and coping with lung cancer. *Western Journal of Nursing Research, 9*, 29-42.

Seligman, M.E.P. (1975). *Helplessness: On depression, development, and death.* San Francisco: Freeman.

Selye, H. (1956). *The stress of life.* New York: McGraw-Hill.

Shillinger, F.L. (1983). Locus of control: Implications for clinical nursing practice. *Image, 15*(2), 58-63.

Singer, J.E. (1984). Some issues in the study of coping. *Cancer, 53*, 2303-2313.

Smith, R.A., Wallston, B.S., Wallston, K.A., et al (1984). Measuring desire for control of health care processes. *Journal of Personality and Social Psychology, 47*, 415-426.

Stoner, M.H. (1982). *Hope and cancer patients* (Doctoral dissertation, University of Colorado, 1983). *Dissertation Abstracts International, 44*(1), 115B.

Stoner, M.H., & Keampfer, S.H. (1985). Recalled life expectancy information, phase of illness, and hope in cancer patients. *Research in Nursing and Health, 8*, 269-274.

Suls, J. (1982). Social support, interpersonal relations, and health: Benefits and liabilities. In G.S. Sanders & J. Suls (Eds.), *Social psychology of health and illness* (255-277). Hillsdale, NJ: Lawrence Erlbaum.

Taylor, S.E., Lichtman, R.R., Wood, J.V. (1984). Compliance with chemotherapy among breast cancer patients. *Health Psychology, 3*, 553-562.

Tilden, V.P. (1985). Issues of conceptualization and measurement of social support in the construction of nursing theory. *Research in Nursing and Health, 8,* 199–206.

Wallston, B.S., Alagna, S.W., DeVellis, B.M., et al (1983). Social support and physical health. *Health Psychology, 2,* 367–391.

Wallston, B.S., Wallston, K.A. (1978). Locus of control: An important construct for health educations. *Health Education Monographs, 6,* 107–117.

Wallston, K.A., Wallston, B.S., DeVellis, R. (1978). Development of the multidimensional health locus of control (MHLC) scales. *Health Education Monographs, 6,* 160–170.

Wallston, B.S., Wallston, K.A., Kaplan, G.D., et al (1976). Development and validation of the health locus of control (HLC) scale. *Journal of Clinical Psychology, 44,* 580–585.

Weinert, C. (1987). A social support measure: PRQ85. *Nursing Research, 36,* 273–277.

Whelan, J. (1984). Oncology nurses' attitudes toward cancer treatment and survival. *Cancer Nursing, 7,* 375–383.

Witenberg, S.H., Blanchard, E.B., Suls, J., et al (1983). Perceptions of control and causality as predictors of compliance and coping in hemodialysis. *Basic and Applied Social Psychology, 4,* 319–336.

Wortman, C.B. (1984). Social support and the cancer patient: Conceptual and methodologic issues. *Cancer, 53,* 2339–2360.

Zeltzer, L., & LeBaron, S. (1983). Behavioral intervention for children and adolescents with cancer. *Behavioral Medicine Update, 5,* 17–22.

CHAPTER 5

Selection of the Research Design

Frances Marcus Lewis
Mel R. Haberman

The purpose of the current chapter is to introduce descriptive, experimental, and quasi-experimental research designs to the beginning investigator in oncology nursing. There are two parts to the chapter: Section 1 reviews the different types of qualitative paradigms as special cases of descriptive design. Three methods of qualitative inquiry are introduced: phenomenology, ethnography, and grounded theory. Section 2 describes selected experimental and quasi-experimental designs and summarizes the threats to internal and external validity. In both Sections 1 and 2 the rationale and advantages for each design are analyzed in order to aid in their appropriate selection.

Let us begin by considering some common situations with which you might be familiar. Each of these situations introduces a category of research designs that will be discussed in more detail in the text of the chapter.

Both the staff nurses and clinic nurses have observed that family members experience a great deal of stress while waiting in the radiation oncology clinic. The staff want to know what they can do for these family members during the clinic waiting period that would help reduce the family's apparent distress. The staff do not know, however, what the family members are thinking or feeling as they wait in the radiation clinic; they also do not know what the family members know or understand about the radiation therapy itself. A review of the relevant literature reveals that family members may be experiencing existential concerns as well as anxiety related to a lack of knowledge about the procedures or their supportive role for the patient (Lewis, 1986b; Gotay, 1984). Although the clinic and staff nurses are very eager to intervene with the waiting family members, they realize that their interventions would be only partially informed. Instead, the staff identify the need to document the particular concerns their population of family members are experiencing as they wait in the radiation therapy clinic. This causes them to choose a descriptive design.

Consider a second situation. Community home health nurses have informally observed that young adult patients with previous experience with a chronic illness seem to do better psychologically with their initial cancer diagnosis than do patients not previously diagnosed with a chronic illness. A review of the literature on the psychological aspects of cancer suggests that previous experience with another chronic illness may provide a cognitive map with which the newly diagnosed cancer patients can predict, understand, and thereby psychologically control their responses to their current cancer diagnosis. Rather than relying solely on their clinical impressions, however, the community home health nurses decide to examine systematically the relationship between prior chronic illness, predictability, uncertainty, and psychological control in the young adult cancer patients. This leads them to choose a descriptive design.

Let us turn to a third example. A team of hospice nurses developed a cognitive behavioral intervention for their advanced cancer patients to reduce their distress and diminish their pain. Although the team has used the intervention on almost a hundred patients, they have not formally evaluated the effectiveness of the intervention. The intervention itself is well developed and based on an extensive cognitive behavioral literature. The nurses and their administrator have also the ability to randomly assign patients to a treatment or to a control group. The hospice nurses now want to rigorously evaluate the intervention. This leads them to choose an experimental design.

Let us consider a fourth situation. Two different hospitals are using two different methods to teach new staff nurses how to support the family members of dying young children. The nurses are aware of the differences in the programs across the agencies and want to examine whether the two methods of support have different effects on the staff nurses' attitudes and actual behavior with the family members. The two methods are well developed and based on literature about staff nurse attitudes and behavior with cancer patients. All the nurses at both agencies must attend their respective orientation programs; they cannot be randomly assigned to one program or the other. This leads them to choose a quasi-experimental design.

Let us consider one more situation. A team of chemotherapy nurses notice that mothers of children receiving outpatient chemotherapy vary in their ability to impart meaning to their child's disease and treatment demands. Mothers who impart meaning to the experience seem less distressed than mothers who do not. Mothers, for example, who think God is teaching them an important lesson find it easier to cope with the disease demands; mothers who think that the disease is merely an infliction of pain and punishment with no purpose appear to suffer the most. The concept of meaning, however, is only partially developed in the literature and there is extremely limited empirical research on the concept (Haberman, 1987; Lewis, 1983, 1986b, 1987, in press; Stetz, 1986). As a result of this limited concept development, the staff decide to explore systematically the concept of meaning in their clinic mothers by carrying out in-depth interviews; this is a descriptive study.

In the remainder of this chapter we will discuss designs appropriate to the above situations. We begin in Section 1 with a discussion of qualitative paradigms as a special case of descriptive design.

SECTION I:

Qualitative Paradigms

Mel R. Haberman and Frances Marcus Lewis

The purpose of a descriptive design is to document systematically the issues, concepts, ideas, or phenomena under study. It is particularly relevant when little is known about the concepts or their relationship with other variables. Ideally, descriptive studies lay bare the essential components of the concepts or issues under study, including such things as their frequency of occurrence, their relation to demographic or background characteristics, and the essential distinctions about the concept's critical properties or dimensions. From a concept development perspective, descriptive designs ideally precede intervention studies. In a descriptive design the investigator wants to know as much as possible about the concepts or phenomena before manipulating them. Descriptive studies are distinguished from intervention studies in that descriptive studies attempt to document what is, not to manipulate or change it.

Descriptive studies are distinguished by the extent to which the conceptual or theoretical framework is developed before the study or as a product of it. Nonqualitative descriptive studies have a codified conceptual framework in advance of the study. This framework includes, at a minimum, the concepts, and their definitions, according to which data will be obtained in the study. In contrast, qualitative studies have as their purpose the development or evolution of a conceptual or theoretical framework as a product of the study. Although the investigator in qualitative studies is guided to varying degrees by both literature and experience, qualitative studies are highly inductive studies. Discovery characterizes the entire enterprise. The specific framework shaping the study is only broadly informed, not tightly developed at the beginning of the study. In a qualitative study, the investigator wants the concepts to evolve, not to be guided in advance by what she or he thinks are the important or salient aspects of the phenomena under study.

In contrast, nonqualitative descriptive studies are shaped initially by a conceptual or theoretical framework. For example, Lewis' (1982) study of experienced control, which is summarized in the Appendix, is an example of a nonqualitative descriptive study. The concept of experienced control over health is defined in terms of an operant conditioning paradigm emanating from early work by Rotter (1954, 1966, 1975) and later work by Wallston's team (Wallston & Wallston, 1978; Wallston, Wallston, & DeVellis, 1978; Wallston et al, 1976). There is no discovery of the definition of the concept; it is declared in advance of the data collection. The investigator's role in a nonqualitative descriptive study is to document the frequency or pattern of occurrence of the concepts the investigator proposes in advance of the data collection process. The role of discovery is restricted. In contrast, Saunders' (1981) study of bereavement in young widows, summarized in the Appendix, identifies the study's organizing concepts through an inductive process. The three major response patterns of widows that Saunders identified evolved as a product of the data analysis; the response patterns were not identified and defined at the study's onset but rather emerged as a product of the data analysis.

Qualitative paradigms are much more than a research design; instead they represent a perspective on how human beings interact with themselves and with their social environment and are guided by a "world view" (Benoliel, 1984). At the core of this view is the assumption that human beings create personal and social meanings as they transact with their surroundings. Several additional assumptions underlie the qualitative paradigm. These assumptions are summarized in Table 5-1 and relate to the manner in which the qualitative paradigm views the nature of reality, the relationship between the researcher and research participant, and the explicit form of knowledge generated by qualitative research.

The implementation of a qualitative study is always based on a methodological perspective. The investigator may select a single theory or methodological viewpoint to guide the research process or may blend several qualitative approaches into a suitable methodology. As an example of the former approach, Drew (1986) conducted a phenomenological exploration that examined obstetric and gynecologic patients' experiences with caregivers. In contrast, Haberman (1987) merged phenomenology, ethnography, and grounded theory in order to discover the personal meanings leukemic patients ascribed to their illness experience and to their bone marrow transplantation. Each of these modes of qualitative inquiry is now described; key characteristics of phenomenology, ethnography, and grounded theory are summarized in Table 5-2.

Phenomenology
Phenomenology gives description to the experiential world of human beings and to the personal transformations that occur as people move through a lived

TABLE 5-1. ASSUMPTIONS OF THE QUALITATIVE PARADIGM

Assumption	Qualitative Paradigm
The nature of reality.	Multiple views of the same reality exist. Realities are constructed, dynamic, and holistic. In principal only a limited portion of reality can be known. Process, form, and relationship are of primary concern.
The relationship of the researcher to the research participant.	The researcher and participant are interactive, influencing one another in an inseparable dialectic. The researcher is close to the data; the insider perspective.
The possibility of generalization.	Ungeneralizable. Working hypotheses are time- and context-limited and can only describe individual cases and unique situations.
The possibility of causal linkages.	Circuity. All entities are in a constant state of mutual simultaneous shaping, making it impossible to distinguish causes from effects.
The role of values.	Methods of inquiry and data collection are inseparable. Values stem from the researcher, participant, research setting and from the theory chosen to guide the collection and analysis of data.
The role of context.	Phenomena can only be understood in their natural context. Overlapping contexts influence all phenomena.

Adapted from Berman, M. (1981), The reenchantment of the world, *New York: Cornell University Press; Lincoln, Y., and Guba, E. (1985),* Naturalistic inquiry, *Beverly Hills, CA: Sage.*

experience. Investigators often integrate aspects of phenomenology and existentialism into a unified philosophical and methodological research design. According to Watson (1979), phenomenological existential inquiry offers nursing the best and perhaps the only research method for understanding the phenomena of health and human responses to illness. Phenomenology is a powerful perspective to elucidating the experience and reality of illness. In illness situations the phenomenologist describes the unique world that has become a reality for the patient. Emphasis is given to understanding the patient's explicit view of his or her existence and illness situation (Kestenbaum, 1982; Van den Berg, 1955).

As a research method, phenomenology strives to elaborate the basic conceptual foundations of a phenomenon, the salient relationships that are manifested as a part of the phenomenon, and the patterns of action that characterize a particular lived experience. As such, phenomenological inquiry emphasizes the subjective and experiential nature of reality versus its objective and concrete aspects. Gergen (1980) also noted that phenomenology is particularly useful in examining phenomena that are subject to patterns of fluctuation and change, since the method is anchored in the assumption that existing patterns of action can never be assumed to remain stable. Colaizzi (1978) offers a detailed description of the alternative designs that may be used for phenomenological research. In general, phenomenologists use participant observation techniques for data collection and various forms of content analysis as data analytic techniques.

TABLE 5-2. TYPES OF QUALITATIVE DESIGNS

Type	Key Characteristics
Phenomenology	Focuses on the subjective, holistic, and experiential nature of reality; on elucidating basic characteristics of phenomena; and on salient relationships, patterns of action and change that characterize movement through a specific lived experience. Data collection by participant observation, interviews, and personal diaries. Data analysis by various forms of content and thematic analysis.
Ethnography	Focuses on identifying the way of life of a designated cultural group, including the group's beliefs, customs, behaviors, objects, and events, and on the shared knowledge and meanings that underpin a given culture. Data collection by prolonged participant observation, multiple triangulation, key informant interviews, written field notes, and the examination of artifacts and archived documents. Data analysis employs taxonomic and componential analysis to examine linguistic structure and the structure of cultural domains (themes).
Grounded Theory	Focuses on the discovery and generation of parsimonious theory to describe a substantive area of human experience. Processes, relationships and attributes that differentiate comparison groups of primary concern. Data collection by participant observation, written field notes, personal diaries, memoing, and key informant interviews. Theoretical sampling guides data collection. Data analysis and collection proceed simultaneously. Theoretical codes and categories are identified by comparative analysis and serve as the descriptive framework for the grounded theory.

Ethnography

Ethnography is another type of qualitative inquiry. Ethnography stems chiefly from the field of anthropology and from the use of ethnoscience as a method to generate knowledge. Ethnographic inquiry refers to the systematic study of the way of life of a designated cultural group (Aamodt, 1982; Leininger, 1978). Ethnographers make a distinction between emic, or native, points of view and the etic interpretations imposed on the data by the investigator. Ethnography identifies and describes the shared knowledge and meanings that underpin a particular culture. By observing and recording the customs, behaviors, beliefs, objects, and events that constitute a given culture, the ethnographer exposes the meanings these phenomena have to the cultural group under study. For example Swanson-Kauffman (1986) used ethnographic techniques to describe the personal and social meanings ascribed to the experience of miscarriage from the unique perspective of women who miscarried. In conducting ethnographic field research the investigator must abandon rigorous scientific control, adopt an improvisational style to meet unexpected situations in the field setting, and engage in extended periods of participant observation using him- or herself as the research instrument (Agar, 1986). Byerly (1969) described an account of the nurse's role as participant observer.

The ethnographer tries to make sense of a specific cultural phenomenon by examining it from multiple points of view. Multiple triangulation is a specific research strategy used to examine a given piece of evidence from a variety of vantage points (Denzin, 1978; Mitchell, 1986). For example, in describing how patients adapt to an oncology unit, the ethnographer might cross-validate the data acquired from direct patient interviews with data obtained from a formal review of the medical records and from interviews conducted with key informants. These informants might include the patient's health-care providers, close friends, and family members. Ethnography uses a variety of data collection methods and sources, including the use of participant observation as a basis for writing field notes, the examination of cultural artifacts, and the systematic review of archived historical documents. During the data analysis the ethnographer may also examine the linguistic structure of the language of a cultural group. Folk taxonomies may be developed to describe the similar components of a cultural dimension, for instance all the kinds of health literature read by people with cancer. On the other hand, componential analysis is used to identify the contrasts and attributes that define a particular category of cultural meaning. For example, leukemia as an illness offers contrasts in its acute and chronic forms as well as in the age groups that are at highest risk for each type of the disease. Spradley (1980) provides an extensive review of methods for developing folk taxonomies and for conducting componential analysis. He also describes the steps involved in writing up the final ethnographic report.

Grounded Theory

As a method of qualitative inquiry, grounded theory is derived from data that are systematically obtained and analyzed (Glaser, 1978; Glaser & Strauss, 1967). The term *grounded* refers to the discovery of theory from data that are anchored in empirical evidence. Grounded theory can be developed in any substantive area of human experience. Stern (1980) noted that the strongest case for the use of grounded theory is research that examines "uncharted waters" or that seeks to proffer a fresh perspective on an otherwise familiar situation. Grounded theory is particularly suited to distinguishing the social processes, relationships, contingencies, and attributes that differentiate a number of comparison groups. Research that exemplifies the use of this mode of inquiry includes Quint's on the impact of mastectomy (Quint, 1963), Mullen's investigation of life after a heart attack (Mullen, 1978), and Glaser and Strauss's (1965) study on the awareness of dying.

Like phenomenology and ethnography, grounded theory uses a variety of data-generating techniques, including participant observation, written field notes, and structured or semistructured interviews. Interviews are generally tape-recorded and transcribed to provide permanent documentation of the dialogue that unfolds between the participant and investigator. Methodological and theoretical memos are also written as a means of data collection. In general, methodological memos describe the timing or staging of interviews and the decisions made by the investigator at different points in the study. Theoretical memos document ideas gained from a review of the literature and the investigator's efforts to organize and impose a theoretical structure on the data as it is collected.

In grounded theory, data collection and analysis often proceed simultaneously. Data are organized into content categories that describe a specific theme or concept that emerges in the data, such as the specific types of coping responses used by cancer patients in certain situations. Theoretical sampling may be used to gather additional data so that new light may be shed on a conceptual category that needs further elaboration (Glaser & Strauss, 1967). Ideally, grounded theory development is complete when no additional information is obtained from either the data collection or the analysis. In the final step of analysis, the most salient concepts that emerge from the data analysis, often referred to as core variables, are organized into a parsimonious theory that describes the phenomenon under investigation. For example, in an analysis of late-stage cancer patients' experiences with personal control, Lewis, Haberman, and Wallhagen (1986) identified the core variable of biding time with four subconcepts: refocusing control, turning it over, monitoring progress, and waiting it out. Several sources provide an extensive coverage of the data analysis techniques used for grounded theory, including those by Glaser (1978), Glaser and Strauss (1967), Spradley (1980), and Stern (1980).

Disadvantages of the Qualitative Paradigm

There are several disadvantages to the qualitative paradigm. Field-setting characteristics present many threats to the loss of scientific control. For example, interviews may be interrupted by nursing care routines, by family visits, or by periods of nausea. Qualitative research is also expensive to conduct. Data costs for each respondent are usually far greater for the field worker than for a standard survey instrument. Qualitative studies are also time-consuming. Many hours are needed to develop sensitivity to the research setting and to its inhabitants. It is also time-consuming to develop rapport with research participants, to establish an atmosphere in which the participant's perceptions can be explored freely, to examine numerous sources of data for the purpose of cross-validation, and to write, organize, and synthesize field notes. Another disadvantage is the limited generalizability of the research findings. Generalizability is affected by the selection biases that occur with nonrandom sampling, by unmeasured characteristics that exist in the sample, and by the heavy reliance on self-report and participant observation data. An uninformed criticism is that qualitative methods lack reliability, validity, and objectivity. However, significant contributions to improving the rigor of qualitative research have been made recently by Lincoln and Guba (1985) and by Sandelowski (1986). Topf (1986) specifically addresses methods for estimating the reliability of qualitative data. Finally, prolonged engagement and extensive involvement with research participants, field settings, and with data analysis may take an emotional and physical toll on the investigator. Investigators are cautioned to develop and to frequently use strategies for distancing themselves from the research endeavor to minimize burnout.

Advantages of the Qualitative Paradigm

The advantages associated with qualitative paradigms are directly related to the method's relevance for nursing science and practice. Qualitative methods offer nursing an alternative or complementary paradigm to the traditional quantitative mode of inquiry (Cook & Reichardt, 1979; Mullen & Iverson, 1986). Qualitative research is highly sensitive to the patient's perceptions and world view and thereby elaborates the experienced reality of illness and health. Qualitative methods offer an opportunity to examine over time dynamic processes that are not subject to static analysis but, rather, vary and change. Multiple triangulation expands our understanding of the scope and the diverse aspects of a single concept, which might otherwise be too narrowly defined. Understanding patients' unique frames of reference and their belief about health and illness can expand nursing's theoretical knowledge of the factors that influence individuals' adaptations to wellness and illness. By understanding the health practices and values that are indigenous to diverse cultural groups, nursing can design therapeutic interventions that minimize the tendency of health-care professionals to superimpose their practices and values on the consumers of care or erroneously to treat patients as a homogeneous population.

The qualitative paradigm is also beneficial to nursing because it offers a means to investigate both the scientific and humanitarian aspects of nursing knowledge and practice (Benoliel, 1984). Qualitative approaches are particularly suited to investigating many of the dynamic processes that are central to nursing, including adaptation, change, decision making, transition, developmental maturation, social interaction, and holism.

With this introduction to qualitative paradigms as a special case of descriptive design, let us now turn to a discussion of both experimental and quasi-experimental designs.

SECTION II:

Experimental and Quasi-Experimental Designs

Frances Marcus Lewis

Experimental designs serve two purposes: to document the extent to which an observed change was produced by the program or intervention, not an alternative cause, and to document the extent to which the observed change is generalizable to other situations (Cook & Campbell, 1979). The first purpose relates to internal validity; the second purpose relates to external validity. An understanding of the threats to both internal and external validity provides a framework for choosing a particular experi...nental or quasi-experimental research design.

Threats to Internal Validity

Clinicians and investigators alike are interested in knowing whether or not their intervention or program "worked" or achieved an acceptable level of change (Green & Lewis, 1981, 1986). Research designs allow us to answer the question with more or less certainty. Because numerous factors other than the intervention or program may cause the observed changes, research designs can be established that guard against these other possible sources of change. These alternative sources of change are called threats to the internal validity of an experiment or intervention study. Internal validity factors directly affect the observations we make or the information we collect on the subjects' performance or behavior. These alternative sources of effect are themselves factors that are capable of producing outcomes; they compete with the experimental treatment to explain any observed differences. The presence of one or more of these threats challenges the validity of our claim that our experimental intervention caused the observed changes. There are 11 sources of threat to the internal validity of an intervention study, which are summarized in Table 5-3.

As oncology nurses we might want to argue that observed change in a patient or family after our intervention indicates that our intervention "worked" or was "successful." This may be our best clinical impression, but it is not a scientifically informed position. Rather, there may be one or more of the threats listed in Table 5-3 operating that could affect, at least partially, the observed patient outcomes. When we want to know whether our intervention and not something other than the intervention caused the observed outcomes, we are concerned with threats to the internal validity of our experiment. When we are able to argue that the threats to internal validity were controlled, we can place reasonably high confidence in our claim that the experimental treatment, not another cause, produced the observed results.

History. The history of the experimental participants may affect the outcome variables. For example, patients experiencing our intervention might also be participating in a wellness awareness program at work that increases their knowledge level about cancer prevention. If knowledge about cancer prevention is our criterion, or outcome variable, knowledge-level scores will be affected or confounded by participation in the work-site program. We would be in a weak position to argue that our intervention caused the observed changes; it might be that the work-site program actually caused the knowledge changes.

Maturation. The maturation of the experimental participants may affect the outcomes. When people mature or develop during the course of our experimental intervention, we must expect that their maturation, not just our intervention or experimental treatment, caused the observed changes. It is common, for example, for children to become more internalized in their perceptions of control over their health as they grow older (Parcel & Meyer, 1978). These changes are expected as a result of the maturation process, not just because of our intervention. If we observed an increase in internalized control after our intervention with children, we would not be able to definitively argue that our nursing intervention changed the children's behavior. Rather, their maturational processes could have been equally responsible for the observed changes.

Testing. The testing or measurement process itself can cause a reaction in the participants of an experiment. Participants react to being measured or monitored. This reactivity, not our experimental treatment, might cause the observed changes. For example, families interviewed about their own level of functioning and coping at home with cancer might be stimulated to improve their coping and functioning as a result of the measurement process itself. This effect could occur in addition to any effects caused by our experimental manipulation designed to improve family management.

Instrumentation. Instrumentation, or errors introduced in the process of measurement itself, including observer or coder error, can cause effects besides those potentially produced by an experimental intervention. Observers, for example, may record changes when they really did not occur, particularly if the observer thinks that the individual being measured is part of an experimental treatment group. The form of the instrument itself may also cause changes in the desired outcome, even if actual changes did not occur. For example, if response options in questionnaires range from 1 to 5 after the intervention but only range from 0 to 4 before the intervention, increases may reflect an instrumentation threat, not an actual change caused by the experimental treatment.

Regression Artifact. A regression artifact, not the experimental intervention, may cause the observed changes. This threat to a study's internal validity is a result of including people in the study who have extremely low or extremely high scores on the criterion, or outcome measures. These extreme scoring subjects would be expected to obtain scores in the center or mean of the sample, that is, regress toward the mean, at the next time they were measured, even if the program or intervention had no effect. Patients with exceptionally extensive stomatitis undergoing bone transplantation, for example, might be expected to have less severe stomatitis at the second time of measurement even if the protocol for mouth care did not work.

Selection. Selection relates to the differences that exist between the types of subjects or respondents recruited into the experimental group as contrasted with those recruited into another group (Cook & Campbell, 1979). Selection is a major potential threat to internal validity in quasi-experimental designs. It is also possible that selection interacts with maturation, history, and instrumentation to threaten the internal validity of the results.

TABLE 5-3. ELEVEN SOURCES OF THREAT TO THE INTERNAL VALIDITY OF EXPERIMENTS

1. **History**

   Experiences or events in the life of the participants that occur concurrent to the experimental treatment, program, or intervention are possible causes of the observed changes.

   Examples: National media releases by National Cancer Institutes; release of widely publicized lay press articles on cancer therapies; neighborhood surge of antismoking campaigns

2. **Maturation**

   Developmental changes in the participants (emotional, cognitive, or physical) that occur concurrent to the program, intervention, or experimental intervention are possible causes of observed changes.

   Examples: Increased disinterest in or boredom with the program I Can Cope as it evolved; increased self-care practices over time as knowledge and experience with cancer increased; altered locus of control as patients grew older.

3. **Testing**

   Reactivity in the participants as a result of being measured or tested before the actual intervention are potential causes of observed changes.

   Examples: Nurses given a pretest on attitudes on sexuality and the person with cancer demonstrate an increased motivation to reflect more positive attitudes in the posttests; heightened anxiety as a result of pretest measurement may cause nurses to study with extra diligence for the posttest.

4. **Instrumentation**

   Methods of data generation (including measurement process or form of instrument or people administering the methods) are possible causes of the observed changes.

   Examples: Questionnaire forms before and after the intervention are different from each other; interview protocol was altered between pre- and postintervention; different interviewers were used at pre- and posttest.

5. **Regression artifact**

   Sampling of extreme scorers (either extremely high or extremely low scorers) on the criterion or outcome measures are potential causes of observed changes; extreme scorers tend to regress toward the mean.

   Examples: Subjects with exceptionally low cancer knowledge scores would be expected to regress toward higher scores even without intervention; patients with high anxiety scores would be expected to have lowered anxiety scores at posttest even without intervention.

6. **Selection effects**

   (Includes selection–maturation interaction and selection–history interaction) Dissimilarity or nonequivalence between the experimental or treatment group and control group at pretest may account for the observed differences at posttest. Selection bias may also interact with history or maturation.

   Examples: More mature learners are recruited into the treatment group as compared to control group; ethnic minorities are unequally represented in the comparison group; males with prostate cancer constitute the treatment group whereas males with lung cancer constitute the comparison group.

(Continued)

7. **Differential attrition or mortality**

   Rates of dropouts differing between the treatment and control groups may account for the observed differences in outcomes.

   Examples: Male partners drop out of the treatment group sooner than do male partners in the control group; teen-age children of breast cancer mothers stop attending family therapy sessions sooner than do children in the control group.

8. **Diffusion or imitation of treatments**

   The observed effects may be due to contamination between the treatment and the control group; they are no longer unique groups.

   Example: Nurses in one agency in two different nursing units are assigned to treatment and control groups but over the course of the study the control group learns what the treatment group is doing and does it too.

9. **Compensatory equalization of treatments**

   The documented effects are due to differentially allocated resources given to the control group in the attempt to "make up" for the group's assignment to the control rather than to the treatment group.

   Example: Nursing administration offers additional monies to staff an outpatient clinic that was otherwise assigned to a control group.

10. **Compensatory rivalry**

    Observed differences are attributable to accentuated performance by the control group.

    Example: Nurses in the control group act with concerted effort to carry out exceptionally thorough oral care for stomatitis when the experimental group delivers a new oral care protocol.

11. **Resentful demoralization**

    Documented effects are due to the exceptionally negative performance by those receiving the less desirable treatment.

    Example: Patients assigned to a pamphlets-only comparison group for radiation therapy decide to not comply with the recommendations in the pamphlet.

Differential Attrition. Differential attrition, or the different rates with which individuals drop out from the treatment or control groups, may account for differences in the outcome measures even if the intervention had no effect. If older partners of women with breast cancer dropped out at a faster rate from the experimental treatment group than did older partners in the control group, and the experimental group scored higher at outcome than did the comparison group, one would be in a weak position to claim that the observed effects were due to the program rather than to this different dropout rate. It might be that one obtained the results one did because the remaining partners in the treatment group consisted of younger males in comparison with the control partners.

Additional Threats. Four additional threats to the internal validity of an experiment were recently identified by Cook and Campbell (1979): diffusion or imitation of treatments; compensatory equalization of treatments; compensatory rivalry; and resentful demoralization. These last four threats have particular interest and importance for the investigator because they can never be solely ruled out through randomization. Diffusion or imitation of treatments involves contamination between the treatment and the control group. This threat is particularly relevant to the internal validity of an experiment conducted within a setting that allows participants in the treatment group to interact or exchange information with the control group. Participants in one group may learn information that was intended only for the other group. Compensatory equalization of treatments involves some source—most typically administration—giving resources to the control group or otherwise compensating for resources or goods that were held back from that group in contrast to the experimental group. Compensatory rivalry in participants receiving the less desirable treatment involves social competition in which the control group may be motivated to perform in ways that decrease the expected differences between the treatment and the control groups. Compensatory rivalry is sometimes called the "John Henry effect." Resentful demoralization of participants involves a retaliation or an accentuated negative performance by the participants who receive the less desirable treatment. Participants know they are receiving the less desirable treatments and shut down or perform poorly on purpose.

Controlling the threats to internal validity increases the certainty with which we can claim that our intervention or experimental manipulation, not some other cause, produced the documented results. If we also want to argue that the obtained results generalize to other sites or populations, we need to be concerned about external validity.

Threats to External Validity

Even if we successfully control for all the threats to internal validity, we still now need to consider other factors that can threaten the generalizability of our results: these are the threats to external validity. Threats to external validity involve the treatment variable and some other variable (Campbell & Stanley, 1963, p. 16). Increasingly we need to pay attention to external validity or generalizability, not just to internal validity (Lewis, 1986a and c; Cronbach et al, 1981).

There are four important threats to external validity: interaction between selection and treatment, interaction between testing and treatment, reactive situational effects, and multiple treatment or combined effects.

Interaction Between Selection and Treatment. It is always possible that the results one observes are due to the population from which the experimental and control groups were obtained. There is an interaction effect between the subjects selected into the study and the experimental manipulation. This is sometimes referred to as subject–treatment interaction. The uniqueness of the population interacts with the experimental treatment to produce the observed results, but these results would not necessarily occur if the program or intervention were implemented with another population. For example, in the seminal experimental study on continuing education in cancer nursing by Padilla's team, it was possible that the results initially obtained on nurse attitudes and knowledge were attributable to the uniquely motivated nurses employed at the agency in which the staff development program was initiated. If that were the case, the generalizability of the experimental treatment would be threatened. Padilla's team evaluated this possibility by later transporting the continuing education program to additional sites away from the hospital in which the experimental study was first conducted (Padilla, Baker, & Dolan, 1975, 1977).

Interaction Between Testing and Treatment. There may also be an interaction between the testing process and the treatment that could threaten the external validity or generalizability of the results. This threat occurs when subjects have been measured or tested before the intervention and the results occur only if the test is given. This means that the obtained results are generalizable to other situations only when the pretest is administered. This threat to external validity is particularly important when the pretest sensitizes the participants, thus making them more influenced by the program or intervention that follows the pretest. In the multistate continuing education study of cancer nursing intervention led by Hongladarom's team, results could be attributed to the interaction between the pretest and the actual intervention, not just to the continuing education program (Hongladarom, 1983; Hongladarom, Lewis, Landenburger, & McCorkle, 1986).

Reactive Situational Effects. Reactive situational effects include a number of factors that are associated or linked with the experimental treatment itself but are not planned components of the intervention. These situational factors can threaten the external validity or generalizability of the results because they would not necessarily be present in other settings to which we wanted to generalize findings. Categories of situational affects include the physical setting of the experiment, the personality or otherwise unique features of those implementing the experiment, the subjects' awareness of their participation in an experiment, and the newness or novelty of the program. For example, a patient teaching–support program conducted in the homelike atmosphere of a newly designed radiation clinic might cause effects not otherwise obtainable in a more typical radiation clinic with an institutional atmosphere. In another example, a smoking prevention program might achieve higher quit rates in an institution with a smoke-free environment than in an agency that permitted smoking. In still another example, pediatric oncology nurses with training in puppetry and children's theater might obtain results in their children's chemotherapy education program that they would not necessarily obtain when the program was implemented elsewhere by nurses not trained in puppetry. In a final example, a newly devised sociodrama designed to help hospital staff adjust to patients' deaths might produce results in one setting that would not generalize to another setting in which ongoing staff support groups already existed (Lewis, 1977).

Multiple Treatment Effects. Multiple treatment effects threaten the external validity of study results. When participants are involved in more than one experiment or program at the same time, it may be the effects of the multiple programs in combination with each other, not just the program being singled out for assessment, that produces the results. This means that we should not expect a single isolated program to have the same effects as the program in combination with others. For example, multiple treatment effects could occur when newly diagnosed patients are admitted both to a physician-directed education program and to the group-focused support and information program, I Can Cope. If our program obtained the desired results, we could be confident in the results obtained in our setting but we would not be free to generalize our results to other settings that did not have similar simultaneous programs.

Choices of Experimental Designs

Despite the numerous threats to internal and external validity, there really are solid design choices one can make to control for these threats. Some of these designs are easily implemented; some require more administrative control than others. The choice of an experimental design should be based on the ability to control the plausible or most likely threats to internal and external validity relevant to one's setting. Three types of experimental designs that guard against most or all of the threats to internal validity are now reviewed: a pretest–posttest control group design; a posttest-only control group design; and a Solomon four-group design. A clinical trials design is also reviewed as an extension of a true experimental design.

Randomization. Experimental designs are characterized by the *random assignment* of study subjects into either the treatment or the control group. The treatment group is given the experimental intervention; the control group does not receive the experimental intervention. The control group may, however, receive an alternative intervention. By randomly assigning subjects, we increase the probability that both the treatment and the control groups will be similar at the start. This puts us in a firmer position to argue that any observed changes are related to the intervention, not to some alternative cause. Stated in another way, randomization controls for most of the threats to the internal validity of our experiment. Randomization also increases the experiment's external validity by controlling for selection-treatment interaction. Using a conservative guideline, random assignment is an equalizer of groups when there are approximately 100 or more subjects allocated into each group (Green & Lewis, 1986). Randomization is particularly important when the expected results of the intervention are small (Shortell & Richardson, 1978, p. 48). Random assignment or randomization cannot, however, be assumed to equate the treatment and control groups in the case of small samples assigned to each group. In all cases the comparability of the treatment and the control groups should be inspected before beginning data analyses. Comparability of control and treatment groups should never be assumed, even under conditions of randomization.

Random assignment may be made simply by randomly allocating subjects to either the treatment or the control groups. There are advantages, however, in first stratifying the population and then randomly assigning subjects from the various strata to either the treatment or to the control groups. Stratification with randomization distributes the study participants into more equivalent groups at the beginning of the study but requires a relatively large initial population from which to stratify and then allocate subjects.

Pretest-Posttest Control Group Design.   The pretest–posttest control group design involves random assignment of subjects into a treatment and a control group. A posttest is administered at the end of the experimental intervention and at the same time to the subjects in the control group. Extensions of this design include multiple treatment groups and multiple posttests. When there are multiple treatment groups, the subjects are randomly assigned to one of many treatment groups. For example recent work by Dodd (1984), summarized in the Appendix, used a four-group design. In her research, adult cancer subjects were randomized into one of four groups: a group that received drug information; a group that received information on the management of side effects; a group that received a combination of drug information plus management of side effects; or a control group that received informal conversation about disease-related issues.

There are a number of advantages to the pretest–posttest control group design with random assignment. All the threats to internal validity are controlled for. Both the treatment and the control groups are similarly affected by all the threats, thus making the observed differences between the treatment and the control groups a result of the treatment, not the internal validity threat. The design also controls for the interaction of selection and maturation and other interactions that could affect the interpretation of the effect of the experimental treatment.

With the pretest–posttest control group design, the investigator can argue that the obtained results were due to the treatment or experimental manipulation, not to one of these threats to internal validity, because both the experimental and the control group were equally affected. Any differences between the treatment and the control groups, therefore, could not be attributed to one of these internal validity factors. We should note some caveats, however. When observers are used in obtaining data for the pre- and posttests, they should ideally be "blind," or not know which subjects constitute the treatment group and which constitute the control group. "Blind observers" cannot introduce their particular bias into their ratings. Selection is controlled for to the extent that randomization equated the treatment and the control groups at pretest. We can be more certain of this when large numbers of subjects are randomly assigned in contrast to when small numbers of subjects are assigned (Green & Lewis, 1986; Campbell & Stanley, 1963, p. 15).

Note, however, that there is no control for a unique intrasession history in the pretest–posttest control group design. Unique intrasession history means that something unique could happen within any treatment session to produce the obtained effects. Examples of such unique events could include the particularly sensitive or empathic introductory remarks offered by the experimenter or the one-time presence of a rehabilitated cancer patient who introduces a cancer film.

Technically, any time there is a different experimenter there is the possibility of intrasession history confounded with the effects arising from the planned experimental intervention. (See Campbell & Stanley, 1963, p. 14, for a discussion of intrasession history.)

Even though the pretest–posttest control group design handles all the threats to internal validity, it does not handle all the threats to external validity. This design does not control for the interaction of testing and the treatment manipulation. The obtained effects could not generalize to subjects who did not receive a pretest. It is always plausible that the pretest sensitized the subjects to the experimental treatment, thereby interacting with the experimental variable to produce the obtained results. It is also possible that selection interacted with the experimental variable to produce the obtained results. Thus, although selection was controlled for as a threat to the internal validity of the experiment, it is possible that the obtained results are relevant only to the particular population from which the experimental and treatment groups were obtained. The frequency with which this particular threat to external validity occurs varies directly with the difficulty in recruiting subjects into the experimental study. Those subjects who are indeed finally recruited into the study are probably unlike the larger population of subjects to which we eventually want to generalize.

Likewise, we can extend our discussion to include interactions between the experimental treatment and other factors like instrumentation, maturation, and history. It is always possible that the obtained effects are due to the particular instruments used in the study; it is the interaction of the experimental treatment with the particular instrument that produces the results, not just the treatment manipulation itself. Alternatively, it is possible that the results are specific or unique to the sampled participants who were all of a particular age. Similarly, it is possible that the obtained results, while internally valid, may only pertain to the particular historical period in which the study was conducted. Any observed results in smoking cessation programs in the mid-to-late 1980s, for example, may be due to the attention paid to antismoking campaigns by federal policy, the National Cancer Institute, and the National Heart, Lung and Blood Institute, not just to the effects of a particular intervention program at a particular agency or in a particular region.

Posttest-Only Control Group Design. The posttest-only control group design is another sound alternative to the pretest–posttest control group design if the nurse investigator is assured that both the treatment and the control groups are similar or equal before the experimental manipulation. In the current design, subjects are randomized into treatment and control groups but do not receive the pretest before the intervention with the experimental group. Currently this design is underutilized in nursing research but presents a sound alternative. Like the pretest–posttest control group design, this design controls for the same threats to internal validity. It also has the advantage of controlling for the potential interaction of testing with the experimental treatment because it omits the pretest as a source of potential threat to the external validity of the experiment. Campbell & Stanley (1963) even argued that the posttest-only design is usually preferred to the pretest–posttest control group design except when randomization does not equalize the groups.

Solomon Four-Group Design. Although seldom used in nursing research, the Solomon Four-Group Design is a true experimental design that explicitly considers external validity. The design allows the investigator to evaluate both the effects caused by testing and the effects caused by the interaction of testing and the experimental manipulation. Groups 1 and 2 in the design are the same two groups as in the pretest–posttest control group design: there is the randomly assigned treatment group and the randomly assigned control group. Group 3 receives the treatment and the posttest but not the pretest. Group 4 receives only the posttest. All pre- and posttests are administered at the same time for all subjects receiving them.

The Solomon Four-Group Design has two more advantages. It allows the investigator to estimate the combined effects of maturation and history on the outcomes. This is done by comparing the posttest-only results from the fourth group with the pretest results of Groups 1 and 2. The design also allows the investigator to interpret more competently past research in an area which used the pretest–posttest control group design. More specifically, the Solomon Four-Group Design lets one estimate the likelihood that past study results were affected by an interaction between testing and the treatment manipulation (Campbell & Stanley, 1963, p. 25).

Clinical Trials Design. The clinical trials design is merely an extension of the pretest–posttest control group design with the addition of a placebo group, "blinded" subjects, and "blinded" clinical investigators. The study by Bishop et al (1984), summarized in the Appendix, provides an example of a randomized, double-blind crossover design. Subjects were randomly assigned into the treatment or the placebo group, just as they would be in a true experimental design. A placebo group means that the participants in the study received a treatment manipulation in the form of an inert substance that was not identifiable as inert; rather it could easily be assumed to be the experimental substance. Clinical investigators were "blind" in that they did not know which of the drugs was the placebo or the experimental drug lorazepam. Subjects were also "blind" in that they did not know if they were receiving the placebo or the actual experimental drug.

In the study by Bishop's team patients were randomly assigned to one of six sequences of lorazepam (L) or placebo (P) (ie, LLP, LPL, LPP, PLL, PPL, or PLP). To keep the investigators and the subjects "blind" as to their treatment status, all drugs were prepackaged with the drug sequence identified by a code number, not by L or P. These codes were not available to the clinical investigators or to the subjects. The investigators chose three consecutive courses of chemotherapy to evaluate the effectiveness of lorazepam in order to reduce the potential effects resulting from observer bias.

QUASI-EXPERIMENTAL DESIGNS

Sometimes the physical or political reality or resources of a situation do not allow the investigator to randomly assign subjects to the experimental treatment or control group. This was illustrated earlier in this chapter in the example in which nursing staff from two different agencies were required to attend orientation classes at their respective agencies. When random assignment is not possible, quasi-experimental designs are used. Quasi-experimental designs are a great boon to the nurse investigator when better true experimental designs are not possible. Key to the use of quasi-experimental designs is a full appreciation of the threats to validity that these designs do or do not control. Selected examples of quasi-experimental designs follow.

Time Series Design

The key feature of the time series design is the presence of periodic measurements on subjects at numerous times before and after the experimental manipulation (Windsor, 1986; Windsor et al, 1984). New staff nurses, for example, may be evaluated at weekly intervals on their skill at administering chemotherapy drugs. After week six, these same nurses participate in a new training program on intravenous drug administration. Evaluations of skill performance continue as before. The director of staff development is interested in knowing whether the new intravenous training program improved the staff nurses' performance. A time series design would be one viable research design to choose under such circumstances.

The time series design has some inherent limitations because of the threats to internal and external validity it does not control. Its most serious limitation is that it does not control for effects resulting from history. It is always possible, for example, that a concurrent program other than the new intravenous training program caused the observed changes in the skill performance of the staff nurses in our example. If, however, the nurse investigator can systematically argue against and rule out the existence of plausible alternative causes of the observed changes in skill level, the credibility of the results from this design are protected. However, ruling out potential concurrent causes of effects with this design is not easy. The seasoned investigator will probably use this design only when three conditions exist: when the cycle of periodic measurements and experimental manipulation can be repeated with a number of samples and in various settings; when there is no possibility of using a more controlled design; and when periodic measurements will occur anyway. This design capitalizes on them.

Under some circumstances the results obtained from the time series design could be threatened by instrumentation. This seems particularly likely if the measurement procedure involves human judges and these judges are aware of the experimental intervention. Such biased observers might plausibly confirm the presence of changed behavior when it really did not occur; it was merely a function of the observer's expectations (Campbell & Stanley, 1963, p. 41).

Threats to the external validity of the time series design include both selection and treatment interaction and reactive situational effects. The selection–treatment interaction reminds us that results may only obtain for the specific sample measured, not to others.

Nonequivalent Control Group Design

The nonequivalent control group design is the same design as the pretest–posttest control group design considered under experimental designs except that it lacks randomization. In the nonequivalent control group design the investigator takes advantage of two naturally occurring groups, one of whom receives the experimental manipulation, one of whom serves as the comparison group. The absence of randomization means that the experimental and comparison groups do not have preexperimental sampling equivalence; they are not technically the same at pretest. However, the careful selection of the two groups is focused on maximizing the similarity between the two occurring groups. Threats to internal validity are minimized the more similar the treatment group is to the comparison group, determined both by the selection process and the verification of equivalence based on pretest scores. The more similar the experimental group is to the comparison group, the more confidence the investigator can have in attributing effects to the experimental treatment.

When pretest equivalence exists, this design controls for history, maturation, testing, and instrumentation. Both the treatment and the comparison groups would be equally affected by these potential threats to internal validity, and the threats therefore could not account for any observed differences between the two groups.

This design does not control for possible interaction effects between selection and history, maturation or testing. Although Campbell and Stanley argue that such interactions are unlikely, they are plausible in certain situations (Campbell & Stanley, 1963, p. 48). If the experimental group consisted of acutely grieving parents of dead children and the comparison group consisted of parents of children with leukemia in remission, a change in the experimental group could be attributable to a spontaneous change because they were an extreme group; this change could have occurred in the absence of an experimental manipulation anyway. Because the change could be inappropriately taken for an effect of the experimental treatment, potential interaction between selection and maturation represents a threat to the internal validity of the design.

The nonequivalent control group design does not control for a possible interaction effect between selection and maturation, even when the treatment and comparison groups are similar at pretest. In the beginning of the chapter we offered the example of two agencies with orientation programs for teaching nurses how to support family members of dying young children. Suppose that at pretest the nurses at both agencies are similar in their attitudes and behavior. It is always possible, however, that the nursing staff at the experimental agency matures at a higher rate than does the staff in the comparison agency. These differences in maturation mean that observed changes in the experimental group could be inappropriately attributed to the effects of the program rather than to the maturation of the experimental participants. This selection–maturation interaction threatens the internal validity of the design.

The nonequivalent control group design also does not control for regression. If either the experimental treatment or comparison group is chosen because it represented extreme scores, it is always possible that the difference between the two groups is related to the natural shift in scores—spontaneous regression toward the mean—that would have occurred independent of the experimental manipulation.

External validity is also threatened in a nonequivalent control group design by the interaction of the treatment manipulation with testing or selection, or by reactive arrangements. The threat to external validity caused by interaction between testing and experimental manipulation is the same as with the experimental pretest–posttest control group design. The selection–treatment interaction is due to the possibility that the observed effects may be caused by the uniqueness of the respondents selected to participate in our study; such results would not be expected to generalize to other potential participants. Reactive arrangements are also plausible counterhypotheses that would prevent generalizability. Campbell and Stanley suggest, however, that threats resulting from reactivity are probably less frequent with this design than they are in the true experimental control group design (Campbell & Stanley, 1963, p. 50). By using naturally occurring groups, the investigator may be less likely to create a reactive environment that produces the effects.

Multiple-Time Series Design

The multiple-time series design is an extension of the time series design that adds a naturally occurring comparison group. By adding the comparison group, the nurse investigator gains increased confidence that any obtained differences between the treatment and the comparison groups are due to the experimental manipulation, not to alternative sources. This design actually allows the investigator to examine treatment effects in two ways: by comparing the pretreatment measures with the posttreatment measures in the treatment group and by comparing the treatment values with the comparison group values. This design has some distinct advantages: it adequately controls for all the threats to internal validity except the possible interaction between selection and history. It is always possible, for example, that the concurrent context may interact with the characteristics of those selected to participate in the study to produce the observed effects.

The external validity of this design is threatened by a testing–treatment interaction, although this design is usually used in situations in which the testing is carried out as a matter of course or usual practice with participants and is therefore not reactive. The design may also be threatened by a selection–treatment interaction. This is a caution one must always consider; effects may be due to the interaction between the uniqueness of the participants and their particular response to the intervention and would not generalize to other nonparticipants. Reactive arrangements may account for differences, but, again, these are unlikely given the circumstances under which most multiple-time series designs would be used.

The multiple-time series design provides a sound design choice when repeated measures are available anyway and when a similar comparison group can be recruited. It is a design worthy of more attention, even though it is relatively rare in the nursing literature.

Because of the inherent limitations in any single method of obtaining information, a growing body of literature emphasizes the importance of obtaining descriptive information from more than one data-generating method in each study (Mitchell, 1986; Green & Lewis, 1986). Information on self-care obtained through a clinic informant's report, for example, can be complemented by additional information obtained from the patient's self-report questionnaire, through case-intensive interviews, or through direct observation.

SUMMARY

The selection of the research design is guided ultimately by the research question one wants to examine as well as the amount of accumulated knowledge in the area of interest. This means that there is no such thing as the perfect research design; rather, the design should fit the circumstances. The chapter reviews selected research designs that provide the basis for examining phenomena in oncology nursing. The qualitative paradigm as a special case of descriptive study is reviewed. Ethnography, phenomenology, and grounded theory provide the bases for generating data for descriptive work. Both experimental and quasi-experimental designs are reviewed, including the threats to internal and external validity. Throughout the chapter the advantages and disadvantages of each research design are considered.

REFERENCES

Aamodt, A. (1982). Examining ethnography for nurse researchers. *Western Journal of Nursing Research, 4,* 209–221.

Agar, M. (1986). Speaking of ethnography. Beverly Hills: Sage.

Benoliel, J.Q. (1984). Advancing nursing science: Qualitative approaches. *Communicating Nursing Research 17,* 1–8, Boulder, CO: Western Interstate Commission for Higher Education.

Bishop, J.F., Olver, I.N., Wolf, M.M., et al (1984). Lorazepam: A randomized, double-blind, crossover study of a new antiemetic in patients receiving cytotoxic chemotherapy and prochlorperazine. *Journal of Clinical Oncology, 2*(6), 691–695.

Byerly, E. (1969). The nurse researcher as participant–observer in a nursing setting. *Nursing Research, 18,* 230–236.

Campbell, D.T., & Stanley, J.C. (1963). *Experimental and quasi-experimental designs for research*. Chicago: Rand McNally.

Colaizzi, P. (1978). Psychological research as the phenomenologist views it. In R. Valle & M. King (Eds.), *Existential-phenomenological alternatives for psychology*. New York: Oxford University Press.

Cook, T.D., & Campbell, D. T. (1979). *Quasi-experimentation, design and analysis issues for field settings*. Chicago, Rand McNally.

Cook, T.D., & Reichardt, C.S. (1979). *Qualitative and quantitative methods in evaluation research*. Beverly Hills: Sage.

Cronbach, L.J., et al (1981). *Toward reform of program evaluation*. San Francisco: Jossey-Bass.

Denzin, N. (1978). *Sociological methods*. New York: McGraw-Hill.

Dodd, M.J. (1984). Measuring informational intervention for chemotherapy knowledge and self-care behavior. *Research in Nursing and Health, 7*, 43–50.

Donaldson, S., & Crowley, D. (1978). The discipline of nursing. *Nursing Outlook, 26*, 113–120.

Drew, N. (1986). Exclusion and confirmation: A phenomenology of patients' experiences with caregivers. *Image, 18*(2), 39–43.

Gergen, K. (1980). The challenge of phenomenal change for research methodology. *Human Development, 23*, 254–262.

Glaser, B. (1978). *Advances in the methodology of grounded theory: Theoretical sensitivity*. Mill Valley, CA: Sociological Press.

Glaser, B., & Strauss, A. (1967). *The discovery of grounded theory: Strategies for qualitative research*. Chicago: Aldine.

Glaser, B., & Strauss, A. (1965). *Awareness of dying*. Chicago: Aldine.

Gotay, C.C. (1984). The experience of cancer during early and advanced stages: The views of patients and their mates. *Social Science and Medicine, 18*, 605–613.

Green, L.W., & Lewis, F.M. (1981). Issues in relating evaluation to theory, policy and practice in health education. *Mobius, 1*(2), 46–58.

Green, L.W., & Lewis, F.M. (1986). *Measurement and evaluation in health education and health promotion*. Palo Alto, CA: Mayfield Press.

Haberman, M.R. (1987). *Living with leukemia: The personal meaning attributed to illness and treatment by adults undergoing a bone marrow transplantation*. Unpublished doctoral dissertation, Seattle: University of Washington.

Hongladarom, G. (1983). A mobile cancer nursing outreach program: Assumptions and realities. *Cancer Nursing*, 49–54.

Hongladarom, G., Lewis, F.M., Landenburger, K., et al (1986). A community-based cancer nursing continuing education program. In G. Hongladarom & R. McCorkle (Eds.), *Issues and Topics in Cancer Nursing* (77–78). Norwalk, CT: Appleton-Century-Crofts.

Kestenbaum, V. (1982). *The humanity of the ill: Phenomenological perspectives*. Knoxville: University of Tennessee Press.

Leininger, M. (1978). *Transcultural nursing: Concepts, theories, and practices*. New York: Wiley.

Lewis, F.M. (in press). Attributions of control, experienced meaning, and psychosocial well-being in advanced cancer patients. *Journal of Psychosocial Oncology*.

Lewis, F.M. (1987). The concept of control: A typology and health related variables. *Advances in Health Education and Health Promotion, 2*, 277–309.

Lewis, F.M. (1986a, September 26–28). *Beyond technique and technology: Who and what is evaluation to serve?* Paper presented at Society of Public Health Educators National Conference, American Public Health Association National Meeting, Las Vegas, NV.

Lewis, F.M. (1986b). The impact of cancer on the family: A critical analysis of the research literature. *Patient Education and Counseling, 8,* 269–289.

Lewis, F.M. (1986c). Whose responsibility is program evaluation in nursing? In R. McCorkle and G. Hongladarom (Eds.), *Issues and topics in cancer nursing* (251–259). Norwalk, CT: Appleton-Century-Crofts.

Lewis, F.M. (1983, May 4–6). *The concept of personal control: Specification and measurement.* Paper presented at Sixteenth Annual Communicating Nursing Research Conference, Portland, OR.

Lewis, F.M. (1982). Experienced personal control and quality of life in late-stage cancer patients. *Nursing Research, 31*(2), 113–119.

Lewis, F.M. (1977). A time to live and a time to die: An instructional drama. *Nursing Outlook, 25*(12), 762–765. .

Lewis, F.M., Haberman, M.R., Wallhagen, M.I. (1986). How late-stage adult cancer patients experience control. *Journal of Psychosocial Oncology, 4*(4).

Lincoln, Y., & Guba, E. (1985). *Naturalistic inquiry.* Beverly Hills, CA: Sage.

Mendenhall, W., Ott, L., Scheaffer, R.L. (1971). *Elementary survey sampling.* Belmont, CA: Duxbury Press.

Mitchell, E.S. (1986). Multiple triangulation: A methodology for nursing science. *Advances in Nursing Science, 8*(2), 18–26.

Mullen, P. (1978). Cutting back after heart attack: An overview. *Health Education Monographs, 6*(3), 295–311.

Mullen, P.D., & Iverson, D.C. (1986). Qualitative methods. In L.W. Green & F.M. Lewis (Eds.), *Evaluation and measurement in health education and health promotion* (149–170). Palo Alto, CA: Mayfield Press.

Padilla, G.V., Baker, V.E., Dolan, V.A. (1975). *Interacting with dying patients.* Duarte, CA: City of Hope National Medical Center.

Padilla, G.V., Baker, V.E., Dolan, V.A. (1977). Interacting with dying patients. *Communicating Nursing Research, 8,* 101–114.

Parcel, G.S., & Myer, M.P. (1978). Development of an instrument to measure children's health locus of control. *Health Education Quarterly, 6*(2), 149–159.

Quint, J. (1963). The impact of mastectomy. *American Journal of Nursing, 63,* 88–92.

Rotter, J.B. (1954). *Social learning and clinical psychology.* Englewood Cliffs, NJ: Prentice-Hall.

Rotter, J.B. (1966). Generalized expectancies for internal versus external control of reinforcement. *Psychological Monographs, 80* (609), 1–28.

Rotter, J.B. (1975). Some problems and misconceptions related to the construct of internal versus external control of reinforcement. *Journal Consulting and Clinical Psychology, 43*(1), 56–67.

Sandelowski, M. (1986). The problem of rigor in qualitative research. *Advances in Nursing Science, 8*(3), 27–37.

Saunders, J.M. (1981). A process of bereavement resolution: Uncoupled identity. *Western Journal of Nursing Research, 3*(4), 319–336.

Shortell, S.M., & Richardson, W.C. (1978). *Health program evaluation.* Saint Louis: Mosby.

Smith, H.W. (1975). *Sampling: The search for typicality in strategies of social research.* Englewood Cliffs, NJ: Prentice-Hall.

Spradley, J. (1980). *Participant observation*. New York: Holt, Rinehart & Winston.

Stern, P. (1980). Grounded theory methodology: Its uses and processes. *Image, 12*(1), 20–23.

Stetz, K.M. (1986). *The experience of spouse caregiving for persons with advanced cancer.* Unpublished doctoral dissertation. Seattle: University of Washington.

Swanson-Kauffman, K. (1986). A combined qualitative methodology for nursing research. *Advances in Nursing Science, 8*(3), 58–69.

Topf, M. (1986). Three estimates of interrater reliability of nominal data. *Nursing Research, 35*(4), 253–255.

Van den Berg, J. (1955). *The phenomenological approach to psychiatry*. Springfield, IL: Chs. C. Thomas.

Wallston, B.S., & Wallston, K.A. (1978). Locus of control and health: A review of the literature. *Health Education Monographs, 6*(2), 107–117.

Wallston, K.A., Wallston, B.S., DeVellis, R. (1978). Development of the multidimensional health locus of control (MHLC) scales. *Health Education Monographs, 6*(2), 160–170.

Wallston, B.S., Wallston, K.A., Kaplan, G.D., et al (1976). Development and validation of the health locus of control (HLC) scale. *Journal Consulting and Clinical Psychology, 44,* 580–585.

Watson, J. (1979). *Nursing: The philosophy and science of caring*. Boston: Little, Brown.

Windsor, R.A. (1986). The utility of time series designs and analysis in evaluating health promotion and education programs. *Advances in Health Education and Promotion, 1,* 435–465.

Windsor, R.A., Baranowski, T., Clark, N., et al (1984). *Evaluation of health promotion and education programs.* Palo Alto, CA: Mayfield Press.

CHAPTER 6

Definition of the Research Variables

Jan Atwood

The purpose of this chapter is to address key issues about data in oncology nursing research. The type and content of a research question or hypothesis directs the rest of the research process. The research question or hypothesis determines the design, the methodology or measurement tools needed, the data to be gathered, and analyses to be done. Thus, the first issue considered here is the types of research questions addressed in oncology nursing research and how they fit with the cancer problem. The second is the match among the research question or hypothesis, the design, and methodology. Appropriate use of qualitative and quantitative methodologies is considered with examples from oncology nursing research literature. Special attention is paid to independent, dependent, and extraneous variables, plus validity and reliability of instruments. Emphasis is placed on practicality issues of sample size, soundness and testing of instruments, standardization of protocols, project facilitation, accessibility of data, and sources of data.

TYPES OF CANCER QUESTIONS ADDRESSED

The American Nurses' Association (ANA) Social Policy Statement (1983) identifies the purview of nursing. Clearly, nursing practice, including oncology nursing practice, includes the three levels of prevention (Leavell & Clark, 1965).

Primary prevention is a strategy of intervention for eliminating symptoms before they occur. Behaviors that prevent cancer are included here, such as particular eating patterns (Kulbok, 1985). Secondary prevention is promotion of early diagnosis and treatment, with a focus on cure. Reduction of physical symptoms such as nausea and vomiting in patients receiving chemotherapy has been addressed by Bishop et al (1984), Dodd (1984), and others. Tertiary prevention aims to prevent further deterioration and to promote rehabilitation, with an emphasis on care rather than cure. Tertiary prevention has been addressed by researchers such as Martinson, Palta, and Rude (1978) in their work with children who have chosen to die at home and the nurses who work with the families. Each level of prevention includes not only physical but psychological aspects of care for patients, nurses, and family members, many of whom are informal caregivers. Lewis (1982), Padilla, Baker, and Dolan (1977), and others have addressed such research questions. In oncology nursing practice all three levels of prevention need a firm research base. Research in the area of primary prevention is an especially high priority, as indicated by the National Cancer Institute's goal of markedly reducing the incidence of cancer in the foreseeable future and by the global World Health Organization goal of Health for All by the Year 2000. Research provides direction for practice, education, and administration.

MATCH AMONG THE RESEARCH QUESTION OR HYPOTHESIS, DESIGN, AND METHODOLOGY

Key features of the research question or hypothesis determine the type of design and methodology used and, subsequently, the data that are generated. These key features of the research question or hypothesis include the degree to which the phenomenon is understood, the maturity of the scientific research base for the research question, and the degree to which instrumentation has been developed to address the question. If the phenomenon for study is not well known, a conceptual perspective or a targeted research question itself guides the study. However, if the phenomenon is well known, very specific, testable research hypotheses can be generated, and they guide the study. The key features of the question or hypothesis impact upon the types of data gathered in the following ways. If a phenomenon is well understood, that means its name and its definition are known (eg, chemically induced alopecia). The research design can be strong (eg, experimental rather than descriptive), the methodology can be sophisticated, and the data from research on phenomena such as chemically induced alopecia are likely to be numerical and replicable. However, if the nature of the phenomenon is obscure (eg, behavioral antecedents to colorectal cancer) the researcher must first discover what the antecedents are and how they are defined. Thus, the design must be more descriptive and the methodology probably inductive rather than deductive. Early data are likely to be qualitative.

The second feature of the research question or hypothesis is the maturity of the scientific base. The more extensive and accurate the research base is in the content areas of the research question, the more appropriate is a deductive design yielding mostly quantitative, statistically powerful data to answer the question.

Third, if instruments (eg, machines, questionnaires) do not exist to measure the variables in the research question or hypothesis, the study design must include developing the instruments and then generating validity and reliability assessment data before the research question can be addressed. Deductive experimental and quasi-experimental designs are the more traditional types. They are characterized by starting with a definitive idea about how variables are related and embodied in a research question that provides the context for the specific research hypotheses to be tested. These determine the data collection methodology used to generate the data. Usually, more quantitative data (numbers) than qualitative (eg, words, pictures, sounds) are produced in deductive designs. In contrast, inductive designs emerge from more general research questions and require the researcher to start with data that are usually qualitative in nature, then to discover the variable labels, definitions, and the relationships among them. Grounded theory strategies are an example of an inductive design.

Philosophers of science have made a major contribution to research across all fields of science by focusing on the degree of understanding that we have about various phenomena. Dickoff, James, and Weidenbach (1968) portray degree of understanding and levels of theory. At the most basic level (Level 1), the research focus is on discovering what concepts or variables are involved in a phenomenon, their names, and clear definitions for them. No research hypothesis is involved. For example, Aamodt's work (1972) with pediatric oncology patients and their families has specialized in exploring what phenomena are and how they are defined. To discover how siblings take care of the child with cancer while the patient is undergoing active treatment, siblings were asked what they do for their brother or sister with cancer. The children replied very clearly and simply with responses such as, "play with him," "clean her room," "not give her a hard time." The result of the research was a taxonomy of ways siblings care for siblings with cancer and undergoing chemotherapy. When too little is known about the phenomenon to generate meaningful deductive questions whose variables could be validly indexed by means of a structured methodology, an inductive methodology is appropriate. Identifying and defining the most relevant variables to study constitute the crucial process of reducing specification error. However, specification error reduction involves not only identifying and defining the relevant variables but also proposing their appropriate relationship to one another. The remaining levels of theory concentrate on the latter but depend on the existence of information about which variables to choose and how they are defined.

The next level (Level 2) involves situation-relating questions. In this circumstance, the concepts or variables have been identified, named, and defined. The purpose of the research is to describe the relationships among the variables.

The question from the Lauer, Murphy, & Powers (1982) study, in which nurse and patient perceptions of the cancer patient's learning needs are identified, uses a descriptive design (Brink & Wood, 1983).

Level 3 is situation-relating and has two degrees to it. Both involve definitive, testable research hypotheses. The first involves a correlational prediction in which two or more concepts or variables are related to each other in a more or less symmetrical fashion. An example of a research question that fits this mode is the Lewis (1982) study in which personal control is related to variables such as quality of life. The second degree of situation-relating research involves a causal relationship; there is a time lag between the concepts or variables so that the one that occurs first is purported to be at least a precursor, if not a cause, of the one or ones that occur second. Examples of such questions are the Kennedy et al (1983) and the Jones and Dean (1980) research on chemocap and the scalp caps, in which application of the scalp caps to prevent hair loss in chemotherapy patients was queried. Research questions can be raised in this mode when the concepts are known, well defined, their relationships have been described, and the focus is on creating explanations for occurrences. In this case, deductive methodologies in a highly quantitative mode are appropriate. A key characteristic of strong oncology nursing research is a deliberate, definitive, informed match among the research question, its conceptual framework, the design selected, and the methodology for acquiring meaningful data.

Qualitative Issues and Examples

Each scientific community experiences historical stages of valuing quantitative methodology over qualitative methodology early in the development of the discipline. It is increasingly apparent in oncology nursing research that the inductive, more qualitative methodologies are needed for research questions in the lesser-known areas of oncology nursing and the field of oncology in general; whereas, the deductive methodologies yielding more quantitative data are appropriate for better-known areas (Atwood, 1984; Brink & Wood, 1983; Glaser & Strauss, 1967; Mullen & Reynolds, 1978; Spradley, 1972). Considerations in the use of a given methodology and the subsequent production of qualitative data include a precise match of the design with the research question, attention to the scientific rigor of the method chosen (eg, constant comparative analysis in the grounded theory methodology), and clear identification and reduction of error sources in the process of data collection.

In the grounded theory method, as referred to in Quint's (1966, 1967) research with dying patients and the nursing staff, careful attention was paid to retaining meaning in the emic data gathered from the patients. The constant comparative analysis method mandates the concurrent coding of inductive data into increasingly refined categories with clearly generated definitions (Glaser, 1978; Glaser & Strauss, 1967). The relationships among the categories ultimately describe a social process, as in the case of Quint's research. Saunders (1981) used serial interviews to identify aspects of bereavement resolution. In addition to careful coding, Saunders used a panel of experts who were widows to estimate the validity of the categories she had identified, such as "uncoupled identity" (Saunders, 1981, p. 323). Other inductive and descriptive deductive methodologies similarly yield qualitative data that may come in the form of words or even pictures (Aamodt, 1972; Brink & Wood, 1983; Field & Morse, 1985). Regardless of the source of the data, strategies to reduce error in qualitative data include careful attention to the methodology and to preserving the emic meaning of the information as viewed by the subjects of the research.

Quantitative Issues and Examples
Descriptive and explanatory research (Levels 2 and 3) require primarily quantitative data (Brink & Wood, 1983). Key issues in the generation of quantitative data focus on clarifying the operational from the conceptual definition of each variable, the independent, dependent, and extraneous variables.

Operational versus Conceptual Definition. The conceptual definition of personal control (Lewis, 1982) covers the broad spectrum of actions that can be taken in response to what happens in life; it is inclusive of that concept and excludes other concepts. Lewis (1982) specified the conceptual definition in operational form so that clear, definitive measurement could occur. Operational definitions are the observable measures for a verbal, conceptual definition (Waltz, Strickland, & Lentz, 1984). There are many operational definitions for any given concept. The choice of a particular operational definition determines the portion of the concept to be captured in a given study. Regardless of how the choice is made, the operational definition is based on the conceptual definition. In the Lewis (1982) study, personal control was operationalized in terms of health locus of control via the Wallston and Wallston (1978) Health Locus of Control Scale plus a single-item indicator of the degree to which life is in the control of the patient (Lewis, 1982). Thus, two indicators were used to operationalize the same concept. Even though one indicator only is often used, at least one measure that represents the conceptual definition of each variable in the study is required.

Independent Variables. In descriptive studies that yield quantitative data, manipulation of the independent variable is not a primary issue. However, for quasi-experimental and experimental studies in which causes, or at least antecedent variables, are of primary interest (Level 3), the independent variable must change or vary and, if possible, be manipulated. Since experimental design is the strongest design, it is highly desirable when a field setting permits it. However, manipulating the independent variable is not always feasible. Experimental designs involve random assignment of subjects to the independent variable and a minimum of two contrast groups (experimental and control), which are measured before and after the independent variable occurs for the experimental group or groups. Quasi-experimental designs lack one or more of these features (Wooldridge, Skipper & Leonard, 1978). For example, we cannot randomly assign who is going to smoke and thus be at high risk for cancer and heart disease. Therefore quasi-experimental designs are appropriate for many circumstances in which experimental designs are not feasible or are simply unethical. Whether a quasi- or true experimental design is used, variability in the independent variable is imperative and needs to be measured.

Validating the Manipulation of the Independent Variable. In an experimental or quasi-experimental design, it must be established that the independent variable is, in fact, being manipulated. Strong designs include pilot testing of that manipulation. For example, in a study testing the effects of a staff education program on nurse and patient outcome, Padilla, Baker, and Dolan (1977) conducted an initial quasi-experimental study in a single institution before the staff development program was transferred to other hospitals in the same geographic area. In fact, the results of the initial study provided sufficient encouragement for other studies to follow.

Dependent Variables. Like independent variables, dependent variables must vary (Wooldridge, Skipper, & Leonard, 1978). Dependent variables change as a consequence of the independent variable in experimental and quasi-experimental studies. They are the subsequent variables, or those that occur later in time than independent variables but are not known to be causally related in descriptive studies. The measurement instruments must be sensitive enough to document the variation that occurs.

Extraneous Variables. Measurement of independent and dependent variables is a minimal requirement for clinical nursing research. However, because field conditions under which oncology nursing research is conducted are often fraught with extraneous variables, a discussion of extraneous variables is in order. Some extraneous variables are under experimenter control and some are not. Two primary strategies are available for handling extraneous variables. The first is identifying the most dominant extraneous variables and controlling them, either by random assignment, matching, or a similar means (Wooldridge, Skipper, & Leonard, 1978). The second strategy is specifying and measuring key extraneous variables that are not under experimenter control. In this way, they can be accounted for statistically. Examples of extraneous variables in oncology nursing research include age, stage of illness, ability with language, and gender. In the Dodd (1984) study of knowledge and self-care behaviors for chemotherapy patients, the extraneous variables were controlled by setting the participation criteria at a minimum age of 18 and an ability to understand English. In the Lauer, Murphy, and Powers (1982) study, only patients on medical-surgical units were included to decrease confounding from intensive care. As indicated earlier, the research focus was the relationships between nurse and patient perceptions of patient needs. In the Bishop et al (1984) study, only adult patients were accepted to reduce confounding from developmental staging. The relationship of interest was the degree to which lorazepam was related to control of nausea and vomiting in patients receiving chemotherapy. In the Padilla, Baker, and Dolan (1977) study, staff were randomly assigned before the program to either an experimental or a control condition to interrupt any direct relationship between the independent variable, the staff education program, and the dependent variables of nurse and patient outcomes.

Measurement Scales (Nominal, Ordinal, Metric [Interval-Ratio]). All variables are measured on some scale. Traditionally, scales have been described in terms of nominal, ordinal, interval, and ratio levels of measurement. However, for practical purposes the last two are being summarized as metric, to identify the characteristic of equal intervals between points on the scale, but without having to make the distinction of whether or not the zero point is arbitrary. As described in Polit and Hungler (1983), the *nominal,* or simplest, level involves identifying categories. The numbers assigned to the categories (1,2,3,4,5) simply distinguish one category from another and have no inherent order. The classification rules state that all items in the same category must have the same number, no two categories may have the same number, and the categories must be mutually exclusive and exhaustive so that each item fits in one but only one category. *Ordinal* measurement accomplishes what its name implies, setting order. One number is larger or smaller than the next, so that their size determines their order, but it is not possible to identify how much larger or smaller. The ordinal level of measurement includes all the features of the nominal level but adds information about one number being higher or lower, larger or smaller, than the next. The *metric* level of measurement includes the characteristics of both the nominal and the ordinal levels with the added information that the space between one measurement "category" and the next is identified as equal. Thus, the difference between a scale point of 2 and 3 is exactly the same as the difference between a 6 and a 7. In oncology nursing research, nominal measurement is found in descriptions of various ways patients take care of themselves to prevent nausea, for example. One approach to care may be no better or worse than the next, but rather, each is different. Independent variables are frequently dichotomous (ie, treatment or none). Ordinal measurement, on the other hand, is encountered in levels of teaching strategies. One strategy may be providing an information booklet about breast self examination; the next strategy may be providing the booklet plus seeing a movie of the examination being performed. The next level of teaching may be the booklet, seeing the movie, and having a return demonstration with a nurse. In this example, each level of treatment is more powerful than the one below it, but there is no way of telling if one is twice as good or three times as good as the one before it. On the other hand, metric measurement is encountered in the doses of antiemetic drugs prescribed.

The significance of identifying levels of measurement is twofold. First the highest level of measurement possible is used to promote accuracy and sensitivity. Accuracy is the ability to capture the entity in measurement and sensitivity is the ability to make fine distinctions from one measure to the next. Precision, on the other hand, is the ability to make that discernment time after time after time. Accuracy is validity and precision is reliability. The level of measurement determines which statistical procedures are appropriate to use.

Instrumentation. Several types of scaling methodologies are readily usable in oncology nursing research. Examples used here are the Likert or a similar type of rating scale, Guttman scaling, magnitude estimation, and visual analogue. The Likert type of rating scale provides a summated rating of the respondent's attitude or rating on a given variable. For example, the Patient Satisfaction Scale designed by Risser (1975) is based on a five-point rating scale ranging from "strongly agree" through "uncertain" to "strongly disagree." The scale consists of three subscales: technical–professional, trusting relationship, and education. After the patient responds to all 25 items in the scale, the items are sorted out by subscale and the patient's score is added up to indicate the patient's degree of satisfaction with the three aspects. Thus, the name "summated rating scale" is derived. Likert-type scales are usually readily designed, fairly easy for patients to respond to, and amenable to achieving reasonable validity and reliability.

Guttman scales are often used in achievement orientation with patients. The Guttman scale involves a technique by which, once the respondent answers negatively to one item on the scale, all subsequent items on the scale will elicit a negative response. For instance, if the scale were indexing manifestations of nausea, the scale is constructed so that each symptom is more extreme than the previous one (eg, anorexia, nausea, emesis). Thus, if the first symptom is not present, the others are unlikely to be noted (Polit & Hungler, 1983, pp. 330–331).

Magnitude estimation is a ratio level technique by which stimuli, instead of people, are scaled (Stevens, 1957). In a study evaluating a change from a mixed to an all-RN staffing pattern, magnitude estimation was used to index the level of quality of care provided by the nursing staff (Hinshaw, Scofield, & Atwood, 1981). For example, the staff estimated the degree to which their colleagues showed competency in technical skills and several other dimensions of quality of care.

Visual analogue scaling is becoming increasingly popular, especially with special patient groups. For example, especially ill or elderly patients respond well to the visual analogue scaling technique of placing a mark along a line that measures the magnitude of a variable. For instance, a patient may be asked to place a mark on a line that indicates how much pain he feels or how nauseated he feels or how effective he believes his antinausea techniques are. MacCrae et al (1984) have used this technique successfully in a colon cancer prevention study.

A variety of scaling methodologies is available to oncology nurse researchers. Basic principles guiding the selection of a particular methodology include its ability to tap the variables being measured, the ability of the respondents to use it, the availability of valid and reliable instrumentation using a given methodology, and the resources available to the researchers to handle the data once they are gathered.

The two key issues in measuring variables include minimizing specification error and minimizing measurement error. Specification error is the error that occurs when a concept is being operationalized, and measurement error occurs in the actual measurement of the variable. Specification error has been addressed earlier in the match between the conceptual and the operational definitions. Validity is the issue. Measurement error focuses primarily on reliability, which includes both the validity and the errors in measurement (Kerlinger, 1986). Several basic validity and reliability considerations need to be made, regardless of the type of instrument being used.

Reliability. Reliability concerns repeatability and internal homogeneity of measures. Two primary issues include: internal consistency and stability of the measure. As illustrated in the testing of the Patient Satisfaction Instrument (Hinshaw & Atwood, 1982a; LaMonica et al, 1986), internal consistency is the degree to which all of the items in a given measure are measuring the same thing, whatever that happens to be. Common coefficients for estimating internal consistency include KR20, KR21, split-half reliability with or without Spearman-Brown correction, and alpha and theta (Anastasi, 1981; Kerlinger, 1986; Nunnally, 1978; Waltz, Strickland, & Lenz, 1984; Zeller & Carmines, 1980). Basic measurement texts consider the calculations for the various types of estimates; however, attention needs to be paid to when a type of estimate should be used. When matched with their respective assumptions about level of data, item difficulties and so forth, KR20, KR21, and split-half reliability (usually with Spearman-Brown correction) are used with shorter tests or where a computer is not available. Alpha is used with unidimensional scales or subscales of five or more items when a computer is available (ie, when items are expected to be parallel to each other). Theta is used when an index is not best described by a single dimension. Theta is computed from the Eigenvalue in a principal components analysis (Armour, 1974). Factor analysis can assist with reliability estimates as well. Confirmatory factor analysis is used to identify the internal consistency of the group of items in a scale or subscale. If the Eigenvalue exceeds 1.0 and each item has a factor loading of at least .400 (Kerlinger, 1986), the items are judged to have internal consistency. In contrast, exploratory factor analysis allows the researcher to identify the underlying structure of an instrument by noting the number and nature of the factors emerging (Nunnally, 1978). However, exploring a predicted relationship like this and comparing it with the substantively meaningful, predicted structure is construct validity rather than reliability.

Stability is the type of reliability involved in the repeatability of measurements from one testing episode to another. The test-retest correlation is one common index of stability (Waltz, Strickland, & Lenz, 1984). Stability is desirable in an instrument when the underlying variable is stable. For instance, trait anxiety is expected to be similar from one week to the next; however, state anxiety is expected to change with the circumstances. Thus, measures of trait anxiety would be expected to be stable from one time to the next; however, state anxiety measures would not. Other forms of reliability that are applicable to selected aspects of oncology nursing research include alternate forms of an instrument. For instance, if the same measure must be given to a patient repeatedly, eventually the patient may memorize the questions and respond as on previous occasions from memory instead of according to present circumstance. In this case, either parallel or alternate forms may be used. Parallel forms index exactly the same content with slightly different questions. Alternate forms also have different questions and they test the same content domain but not exactly the same aspects of it.

Other types of reliability that are commonly indexed in oncology nursing research are interrater and intrarater, intercoder and intracoder reliability. Each time the data change form, a reliability check is appropriate. For example, if a patient is observed in a self-care behavior, the information changes from a behavior to a check mark on a code sheet. A reliability check from one rater to the other for the same observations is advisable during a training session. This is interrater reliability. In addition, consistency within each rater from one rating to the next must be trained to standard and assessed (intrarater reliability). If the check marks on the page are transferred into a computer by coders, the data have changed form once again. Another reliability check is in order, both intracoder (within each coder) and intracoder (between coders). Criteria for how much is enough in reliability are available (eg, Atwood 1980; Nunnally, 1978).

Validity. Validity is the degree to which truth or the actual value on a variable is captured (Nunnally, 1978). Validity is really the link between the conceptual and the operational definition of a variable. The better the match, the better the validity. Face, content, criterion, construct validity, contrast groups, and theoretical modeling are applicable validities to consider.

Face validity is the degree to which an instrument appears to measure what it is purported to measure. For example, in the Patient Satisfaction Scale, Risser (1975) designed the scale in such a way that the items appear to measure patient satisfaction. Content validity is usually assessed by a panel of judges. The judges are experts in the area under study. For instance, one appropriate panel of judges for the Patient Satisfaction Scale would be the patients themselves. The judges would be asked to indicate for each item whether or not they felt the item measured patient satisfaction and specifically to which subscale it belonged. A second example is the panel of three nurse experts in oncology patient teaching who were asked to independently judge the representativeness of the learning needs questionnaire items in the Lauer, Murphy, and Powers (1982) study. The questionnaire was designed to identify the learning needs of cancer patients as perceived by the patients themselves and a comparison group of nurses.

Criterion-related validity is the degree to which an instrument of interest correlates with a known instrument validly measuring the variable under consideration. For example, with the Patient Satisfaction Scale, patients' responses on the new Patient Satisfaction Scale could be correlated with their responses on a patient satisfaction scale known to be valid and reliable, if there were one. The higher the correlation, the higher would be the criterion-related validity. Criterion-related validity comes in two types: concurrent and predictive. If both measures are taken at the same time, it is concurrent validity. If they are taken at different points in time, it is predictive (ie, one is said to predict the value of the other variable).

Construct validity involves empirically checking out the performance of a scale according to a theoretical prediction and is, therefore, the most rigorous type of validity. Two kinds of construct validity are considered here in addition to the exploratory factor analysis mentioned earlier: contrast groups and theoretical modeling.

Contrast group validity is a method of identifying whether or not a new instrument can tell the difference between groups with different amounts of the concept. For example, the Patient Satisfaction Scale was sensitive to differences in the patient satisfaction at various stages of a change from mixed to all-RN staffing in the All-RN Staffing Study (Hinshaw & Atwood, 1982a).

Theoretical modeling is the most rigorous type of construct validity. It differs from contrast groups by having more than one theoretically predicted relationship to assess and having the context of an entire theoretical model. Construct validity of the Patient Satisfaction Scale was estimated in the context of the Operative Trajectory Study. The theoretical model predicted that patients' satisfaction would be influenced directly by preoperative teaching activities and indirectly by the intraoperative activities that the nursing staff performed (Hinshaw & Atwood, 1982a, p. 175). Multiple regression techniques are used to evaluate the theoretical model using the new instrument. Criteria for how much is enough are available for each of the validity and reliability estimates in such sources as Anastasi (1981), Atwood (1980), Nunnally (1978), Waltz, Strickland, and Lenz (1984), and Zeller & Carmines (1980).

Measurement theory and data analysis technology have progressed to a very sophisticated level. Validity and reliability estimation procedures are possible for instruments used in clinical nursing research. Whether or not the researcher undertakes the program of instrument development or uses an instrument already developed, attention to validity and reliability are imperative for interpretation of the results of the scales.

Sources of Published Scales. Owing to the complexity and time involved in generating instruments, using existing instruments is an efficient strategy. Sources for instruments include compendia such as the *Annual Review of Nursing Research,* the Ward and Lindeman (1979) and Ward and Fetler (1979) compilations of instruments, and research-oriented journals in which validity and reliability testing are reported with increasing frequency (eg, *Nursing Research, Research in Nursing and Health, Western Journal of Nursing Research*). When selecting an instrument, the validity and reliability issues just discussed and the practicality issues below need to be considered.

Practicality Issues

Practicality enters heavily in oncology nursing research. The first practical issue is sample size. Sample size concerns the size of the patient or family member samples as well as the nurse samples. When oncology patients are undergoing active treatment or are in a difficult stage of their illness, there may be a relatively small percentage of the patients seen in a given setting who have the energy or the inclination to be involved in research. In addition, since the patients are compromised because of their disease process, it is vital to achieve maximum power in a research design with the minimum sample size necessary. Thus, soundness of the instruments is important. In fact, valid and reliable instruments are crucial for all types of data required. In terms of nurse samples, a similar limitation of the total number of staff involved in a particular clinic or unit or setting places an upper limit on the number of subjects available for a given study. Of those staff who are employed in a given setting, patient care demands, staffing requirements, and other very practical matters sometimes limit the availability of staff to participate in research. Thus, the data gathering instruments and procedures need to be as efficient, effective, and as appealing as possible to maximize obtaining the most data in the least amount of time. Characteristics of the sample make practical issues imperative. As illustrated in the Padilla, Baker, and Dolan (1977) study, the desirable instrument characteristics include validity, reliability, brevity, ready understandability, ease of administration, minimal use of energy by the patients, and instrument flexibility such that patient selectivity of response does not promote too much missing data for the respondent's data set to be useful (Padilla, Baker, & Dolan, 1977, pp. 103–104).

The second practicality issue is the testing of data collection instruments. For many phenomena in oncology nursing research, there are no instruments existing to measure them. Some existing instruments are not useful for particular populations. Thus, instruments may need to be generated or adapted. Once the instruments are designed to account for validity and reliability, entire programs of research are often required before an instrument is deemed scientifically strong enough to meet validity and reliability standards. A major ethical question is the source of revenue for conducting these studies and how long patients need to wait before benefiting from instrumentation. Programs of research done in the context of other administrative quality assurance and clinical studies, as described in Hinshaw and Atwood (1982a), combine the features of maximizing validity and reliability while effectively conducting hypothesis testing to the degree to which the instruments permit. Simplicity of design for research instruments for clinical use is imperative (Padilla, Baker, & Dolan, 1977). Economic trends and the expectation of scientific excellence require the ultimate in creativity on the part of the oncology nurse researcher in gathering valid and reliable data in the safest, most efficient, effective manner feasible.

Standardization and reliability of the protocol is the third practical issue. Whether the protocol is a formal experiment or a general descriptive one, standardization and reliability of the protocols are imperative. Reduction of such protocol error is standard practice in laboratory procedure (Skoog & West, 1969). However, field protocols require equal attention to this error source. Reduction of protocol error includes setting up the data collection procedures in a meaningful manner, training observers or instrument administrators before beginning the study, pilot testing the protocol, and then doing protocol checks periodically throughout the study, particularly if several months of data collection are involved. For example, in all of the studies used to document the validity and reliability of the Patient Satisfaction Instrument, a protocol was used by the researchers involved (Hinshaw & Atwood, 1982a; La Monica et al, 1986).

The fourth practicality issue is the facilitation or constraint exercised on the current research project as a result of other projects that are being conducted at the same time. A different concurrent study that requires a great deal of response energy on the part of the patient may limit the amount and usability of the data being gathered in the nurse researcher's study. In this case, coordination among investigators and a deliberate strategy of using similar data collection instruments for two or more studies sometimes maximizes the mileage obtained from expenditure of sparse patient energy.

Another issue of practicality is the accessibility of the data. Although it may be desirable to obtain observational data for the patient in the home setting while she or he is implementing teaching that was done or using equipment to which he or she was oriented in clinic, it may or may not be practical to go to the patient's home and conduct the observation. Some clinic market areas encompass hundreds of miles. Some patients do not have telephones, and the feasibility of setting and completing a home visit on the first, second, or third try is marginal. In this case, a recall set of data may be required instead of a direct observation, even though recall data are known to contain more measurement error than reliable, valid observational data.

The last issue of practicality is sources of data. Using existing data sources and instruments is very efficient for the researcher, if the data are available and the instruments are both valid and reliable. In addition, the research findings have a good chance of being used if they relate to other information similarly gathered on an ongoing basis in the setting. An example is the linear self-assessment scale used in the Bishop et al (1984) study of nausea in patients receiving cytotoxic therapy. Scales like this one and the Karnofsky scale (Karnofsky & Burchenal, 1949) used routinely in clinical practice are prime candidates for use in clinical research.

Patient records are another source of data that is readily available, especially to in-house and consortium researchers. With sophisticated strategies evolving for promoting and monitoring efficient health-care delivery systems, patient records contain a wealth of data. For example, nursing care complexity is routinely monitored as a basis for nurse staffing and for billing. Some patient classification systems have been extensively tested and have known high levels of validity and reliability (eg, Hinshaw & Atwood, 1982b). In addition Padilla and Grant (1982) report the integration of research into a quality assurance program with a goal of maximizing patient's self-care effectiveness. Patients' self-report, subjective scale scores can also be related to certain objective laboratory findings to form multiple indicators of variables such as stress and anxiety. However, additional work is needed for the implications of cross-modality multiple indicators to be clear for clinical research. In addition, the same validity and reliability issues applicable to other measures are relevant here and need to be addressed before an existing data set is used.

SUMMARY

The science of cancer prevention and control is characterized by pockets of knowledge and vast areas of the unknown. Deductive research designs yielding primarily quantitative data are appropriately used to address the pockets of knowledge; whereas inductive designs yielding a preponderance of qualitative data are appropriate for lesser-known areas. Careful attention to error reduction strategies is vital in the collection of both types of data. The development of data collection instruments is a series of successive approximations to the ideal levels of validity and reliability. Practicality is vital. Rich reservoirs of existing data provide opportunities for creative research. The complexity of the cancer problem requires that some research questions be addressed by individual disciplines (eg, nursing) and some by multidisciplinary teams.

The bench marks of credible oncology research are strong science, dynamic practicality, meaningful use of resources, and prompt reporting of findings. The many current and future cancer patients and their families are counting on the conduct of credible oncology nursing research.

REFERENCES

American Nurses' Association. (1983). *ANA Policy Statement*. Kansas City, MO: American Nurses' Association.

Aamodt, A. (1972). The child view of health and healing. In M. Batey, (Ed.), *Communicating Nursing Research: Vol. 5*, (38–45) Boulder, CO.

Anastasi, A. (1981). *Psychological testing* (5th ed.). New York: Macmillan.

Armour, D.J. (1974). Theta reliability and factor scaling. In H. Costner (Ed.), *Sociological Methodology* (17–24). San Francisco: Jossey-Bass.

Atwood, J.R. (1980). Development of instruments for measurement of criteria: From a research perspective. *Nursing Research, 29,* 104–108.

Atwood, J.R. (1984). Strategy for theory development: Grounded theory. *Proceedings of First Annual Nursing Science Colloquium* (37–55). Boston, MA: Boston University.

Bishop, J.F., Olver, I.N., Wold, M.M., et al (1984). A randomized, double-blind, crossover study of a new antiemetic in patients receiving cytotoxic chemotherapy and prochlorperazine. *Journal of Clinical Oncology, 1,* 691–695.

Brink, P.J., & Wood, M.J. (1983). *Basic steps in planning nursing research: From question to proposal* (2nd ed.). Monterey, CA: Wadsworth.

Dickoff, J., James, P., Weidenbach, E. (1968). Theory in a practice discipline: Part 1. *Nursing Research, 17*(5), 415–435.

Dodd, M.J. (1984). Measuring information intervention for chemotherapy knowledge and self care behavior. *Research in Nursing and Health, 7,* 43–50.

Field, P.A., & Morse, J.M. (1985). *Nursing research: The application of qualitative approaches.* Rockville, MD: Aspen.

Glaser, B. (1978). *Theoretical sensitivity.* Mill Valley, CA: Sociology Press.

Glaser, B., & Strauss, A. (1967). *Discovery of grounded theory.* Chicago: Aldine.

Hinshaw, A.S., & Atwood, J.R. (1982a). A patient satisfaction instrument: Precision by replication. *Nursing Research, 32,* 170–175.

Hinshaw, A.S., & Atwood, J.R. (1982b). Factors impacting on the delivery of quality nursing care. *Nursing Research, 31,* 120–121.

Hinshaw, A.S., Scofield, R., Atwood, J. (1981). Staff, patient, and cost outcomes of all-RN staffing. *Journal of Nursing Administration, 11,* 30–36.

Jones S., & Dean, J. (1980). Kimo cap [Letter to the editor]. *Oncology Nursing Forum, 7*(1), 7.

Karnofsky, D.A., & Burchenal, J.H. (1949). The clinical evaluation of chemotherapeutic agents in cancer. In D.A. Karnofsky & J.H. Burchenal (Eds.), *Evaluation of chemotherapeutic agents* (191–205). New York: Columbia University Press.

Kennedy, M., Packard, R., Grant, M., et al (1983). The effects of using Chemocap on occurrence of chemotherapy-induced alopecia. *Oncology Nursing Forum, 10*(1), 19–23.

Kerlinger, F.N. (1986). *Foundations of behavioral research* (2nd ed.). New York: Holt, Rinehart & Winston.

Kulbok, P.P. (1985). Social resources, health resources, and preventive health behavior: patterns and predictions. *Public Health Nursing, 2,* 67–81.

LaMonica, E.L., Oberst, M.T., Madea, A.R., et al (1986). Development of a patient satisfaction scale. *Research in Nursing and Health, 9,* 43–50.

Lauer, P., Murphy, S.P., & Powers, M.J. (1982). Learning needs of cancer patients: A comparison of nurse and patient perceptions. *Nursing Research, 31,* 11–16.

Leavell, H.R., & Clark, G.G. (1965). *Preventive medicine for the doctor in his community: An epidemiological approach* (3rd ed.). New York: McGraw-Hill.

Lewis, F.M. (1982). Experienced personal control and quality of life in late-stage cancer patients. *Nursing Research, 31,* 113–119.

Martinson, I., Palta, M., Rude, N. (1978). Death and dying. *Nursing Research, 27*(4), 226–229.

MacCrea, F.A., Hill, D.J., St. John, K.J.B., et al (1984). Predicting colon cancer screening behavior from health beliefs. *Preventive Medicine, 13,* 115–126.

Mullen, P.D., & Reynolds, R. (1978). The potential of grounded theory for health education research: Linking theory and practice. *Health Education Monographs, 6,* 280–293.

Nunnally, J. (1978). *Psychometric theory.* New York: McGraw-Hill.

Padilla, G.V., Baker, V.E., Dolan, V. (1977). Interacting with dying patients. In M.V. Batey (Ed.), *Communicating nursing research: Vol. 8. Nursing research priorities: Choice or chance* (101–114). Boulder, CO: Western Interstate Council for Higher Education.

Padilla, G.V., & Grant, M.M. (1982). Quality assurance programme for nursing. *Journal of Advanced Nursing, 7,* 135–145.

Polit, D., & Hungler, B. (1983). *Nursing research: Principles and methods.* Philadelphia: Lippincott.

Quint, J. (1966). Awareness of dying and the nurse's composure. *Nursing Research, 15,* 49–55.

Quint, J. (1967). *The nurse and the dying patient.* New York: Macmillan.

Risser, N. (1975). Development of an instrument to measure patient satisfaction with nurses and nursing care in the primary care setting. *Nursing Research, 24,* 45–52.

Saunders, J.M. (1981). A process of bereavement resolution: Uncoupled identity. *Western Journal of Nursing Research, 3,* 319–335.

Skoog, D.A., & West, D.M. (1969). The evaluation of analytical data. In *Fundamentals of Analytical Chemistry* (2nd ed.) (25–58). New York: Holt, Rinehart & Winston.

Spradley, J.P. (Ed.). (1972). *Culture and cognition.* San Francisco: Chandler.

Stevens, S.S. (1957). On the psychophysical law. *Psychological Review, 64,* 153–181.

Wallston, K.A., & Wallston, B.S. (1978). Development of the multidimensional health locus of control (MHLOC) scales. *Health Education Monographs, 6*(2), 160–170.

Waltz, C., Strickland, O., & Lenz, E. (1984). *Measurement on nursing research.* Philadelphia: Davis.

Ward, M.J., & Fetler, M. (1979). *Instruments for use in nursing education research.* Boulder, CO: WICHE.

Ward, M.J., & Lindeman, C. (1979). *Instruments for measuring nursing practice and other health care variables* (Vols. 1 & 2) (DHEW Publication No. HRA 78-53). Washington, DC: U.S. Government Printing Office.

Wooldridge, P., Skipper, J., Leonard, R. (1978). *Methods of clinical experimentation to improve patient care.* St. Louis: Mosby.

Zeller, R.A., & Carmines, E.G. (1980). *Measurement in the social sciences: The link between theory and data.* New York: Cambridge University Press.

CHAPTER 7

Analysis of Data

Robert Hill
Gerald Metter

Many researchers think of the need for statistical input only after they have collected a vast amount of data and are at a loss as to what to do with those data. Although this is an important time for statistical involvement, consultation at the time the study is designed is highly recommended. Early statistical input helps to clarify problems in design, define the types of data collected and measurement scales used, plan the types of analyses needed to answer the research question, and determine if the design, sample size, scales used, and analyses planned will, indeed, answer the question.

This chapter introduces some of the basic statistical principles and methods used in cancer nursing research. Considerable emphasis is placed on the logical construct underlying the inferential process and the role of uncertainty. One thing to keep in mind is that results and conclusions should make sense in the context of the research question; even if there are elaborate statistical analyses performed, the end product should make sense. Results will not necessarily be as one might have hypothesized, but they should be comprehensible and reasonable. The overall aim of cancer nursing research is to learn something that is applicable to other similar patients.

DETERMINATION OF REQUIRED SAMPLE SIZE

One of the first things with which a researcher is concerned when designing a study is deciding how many subjects must be included in the study. Often, there are limitations on time and resources that will dictate how many subjects can be included. In such a case, it might not be possible to do the study as planned, and modifications of the design might be necessary. A statistician does not just pull a number out of a magic sample-size-determination hat; the study design and types of data to be collected are critical factors in sample size determination. Virtually every study needs such input, whether it is a randomized double-blind clinical trial comparing two antiemetic drugs or a survey to determine the nursing care needs of elderly patients with ostomies. For these reasons, a statistically unsophisticated investigator should consult with a statistician about sample size and study design.

When asked the question "How many subjects do I need?" a biostatistician will answer with a series of questions: what is the end point of primary interest, how large a difference do you wish to be able to detect between the treatments (or study conditions), approximately how large is the (unknown) population variance of the variable of interest, at what significance level and with what power do you wish to test your hypothesis? (Definitions of significance level and power are given in this chapter, in the section on hypothesis testing.) It may not be easy to answer some of these questions, and an extended discussion may be necessary before the appropriate computations can be performed. The computations do depend on all of those items. Sometimes an investigator will know how many subjects will be available for the study and may want to know whether there will be adequate power to detect a reasonable difference between treatments. Sometimes it turns out that the study is not feasible because the required sample size is too large; in such cases, the investigator may have to redesign the study, decide not to do it at all, or possibly enlist other investigators to join in the study.

The items listed in the biostatistician's list of questions affect the sample size. For instance, the sample size increases as the difference between the two treatments you wish to be able to detect decreases, as the variance increases, as the significance level is made smaller, and as the power increases.

As an example, assume we are comparing midarm circumference in two groups of people. If the variance of midarm circumference is determined to be 2 inches and we want to be able to detect an average difference of 1 inch between the two groups with a significance level of 0.05 and power 0.9, we need to measure 52 individuals in each group. If the difference we wish to detect decreases to ½ inch, we need to increase the sample size all the way to 208 per group. Alternatively, if the variance doubles to 4 inches, the requirement is 104 per group. Decreasing the significance level to 0.01 increases the required sample size to 72 per group. Finally, if we want to have a power of 0.95 instead of 0.9, we must have 62 per group.

BASIC MEASURES—DESCRIPTIVE STATISTICS

Experimental Units

It is important to be clear about the actual experimental unit that is of concern in a given study. In most studies, the individual subject or patient is of interest. However, sometimes we may be interested in studying the family as the experimental unit, or the nursing service, or the hospital, or the health-care delivery system. It all depends on the question being asked, and one must be careful to understand what that experimental unit is, because the analysis of the inferences drawn will depend on it.

Types of Data

Data can come in a variety of types and various names are given to them. The simplest types of data are called *nominal* or *categorical,* and the simplest of these are "yes–no" or "present–absent." Such data are called *dichotomous* and are widely encountered. Another common type of nominal data includes more than two categories. Examples are eye color, diagnostic group, race, occupation, and blood type. No ordering is implicit in the way the categories are listed. Where we have categorical data with ordering inherent, we have *ordinal* data; examples are symptom ratings (0, 1+, 2+, 3+, 4+) and patient satisfaction scores (not at all, a little, very, completely satisfied). The rankings only mean that one category is higher or lower than another; rankings do not mean that categories are equally spaced on a scale.

Another major type of data is measured on scales with equally distant intervals. In one type of scale, an *interval* scale, the zero end of the scale is placed in an arbitrary position. A typical example is the Fahrenheit temperature scale. A *ratio* scale includes equidistant intervals and an absolute zero end point. A typical example is weight.

Data can also be classified as discrete or continuous. *Discrete* data refers to data yielded by counting occurrences of an event, for example, the number of absences from work in a year, the number of children in a family, or the daily number of hospital admissions. *Continuous* data are those measured on an uninterrupted scale such as height, blood pressure, serum cholesterol level, length of time a surgical patient spends in the recovery room, and so on.

Summary Statistics

Graphical Methods. A data set can be summarized in a graphical way using a "histogram," or bar graph, a line graph, or other visual representation of the data. In constructing a histogram for a particular variable, the range of the observed values of that variable is divided into an arbitrary number of subintervals (usually around ten) of equal length; then the number of observations that fall into each subinterval is determined, and a bar is drawn above each with the height of the bar representing the number of observations. The subinterval boundaries should be selected in such a way that there is no ambiguity as to where a value that falls on the boundary should be placed.

A line graph is constructed by making a mark for each subinterval at a height representing the number of observations and connecting the marks with a line to emphasize the changes in frequency from subinterval to subinterval.

Other graphical methods have been developed in recent years, and they are just beginning to gain acceptance in applied areas. These methods often have interesting names such as "stem and leaf" plots and "box" plots. We will not discuss these here.

Measures and Location. Though graphical methods are very useful in providing a quick picture of the nature of our data, we often wish to have one or two "statistics" to summarize the data. The first types of statistics are those that measure location; actually, they measure the middle of the distribution in one sense or another.

The most common measurement is the *mean*, which is just the simple arithmetic average: the sum of the values of the individual observations divided by the number of observations. In mathematical notation:

$$\overline{X} = \frac{1}{n}\left(\sum_{i=1}^{n} x_i\right) = \frac{1}{n}(x_1 + x_2 + x_3 + \ldots, + x_n)$$

where x_i = value of the ith observation, and n is the number of observations. The symbol Σ is the capital Greek letter sigma, and we read it as "the sum as i goes from one to n." This measure is used for interval- and ratio-type data. Since the mean is very sensitive to unusually large or small (so called "outlying") observations, it is typically only used if the data do not include such observations. Data distributed according to the normal distribution, discussed below, provide an example in which the mean is an appropriate measure of locations. Indeed, the mean was developed with this distribution in mind.

The second most common measure of location is the *median*. This is the observation for which half of the observations are smaller in value, and half are larger. To find the median, the observations must be put into order of increasing value; then if n is an odd number, the median is found by taking the $n + 1/2$th observation; for example if $n = 15$, the median would be the $15 + 1/2 = 16/2 = $ 8th largest value. If n is an even number, the median is the average of the $n/2$th and the $n + 2/2$th observation; for example if $n = 10$, the median would be the average of the values of the $10/2 = $ 5th and $10 + 2/2 = 12/2 = $ 6th observations. The median is also most appropriately applied to interval- or ratio-type data. It is, however, much less sensitive to outlying data than is the mean and is a better measure of locations in these areas.

A third measure of location is the *mode*. This is the most frequently occurring value. The mode is typically used for ordinal data. As an example, assume one were looking at the number of male children in families with four children and got the following results:

Number of Males	Number of Families
0	2
1	15
2	47
3	17
4	1

Then the mode would be 2, since it is by far the most frequently occurring value.

For nominal data, a summary measure of location would have no meaning, so none of the three measures given above should be used.

Measures of Dispersion. The second common type of summary measurement measures the dispersion, or spread, of the observed values. The simplest is the *range;* this is the difference between the value of the largest and smallest observations when they are ordered; often, the range is reported as the "smallest to largest" values. The most commonly used measure of dispersion is the variance (and its square root, the standard deviation). The variance, S^2, is the average of the square of the differences between the individual values and their mean; in mathematical notation:

$$S^2 = \frac{\sum_{i=1}^{n} (x_i - \overline{X})^2}{n-1} = \frac{(x_i - \overline{X})^2 + (x_2 - \overline{X})^2 + \ldots + (x_n - \overline{X})^2}{n-1}.$$

We divide by $n - 1$ rather than n for statistical reasons. The standard deviation is more easily interpreted, since it is in the same unit (eg, "inches" in the case of height) as the variable we are observing and it is written as s.

To illustrate dispersion, Figure 7–1 shows two histograms (note that these histograms are laid on their sides and that the frequency in each interval is denoted by asterisks [*] rather than a bar). The histograms both represent normally distributed data with a mean of 100. The one on the right, however, has greater dispersion ($s = 15$ and range = 80) than the one on the left ($s = 10$, range = 50).

ESTIMATION

Population Versus Sample

Much of statistics is concerned with trying to learn something about a large group from a small sample that is representative of that group. Among the most familiar situations is the survey sample exemplified by the Gallup Poll. A typical survey would sample 1200 voters to determine how they will vote in an upcoming election. In that case, the population of interest (which could be a city, state, or

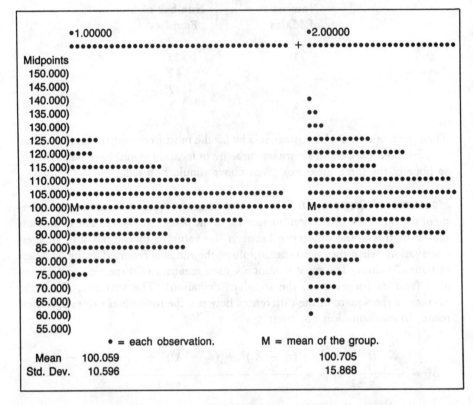

Figure 7-1. Two histograms of normally distributed data.

the whole country) is the voting public in the jurisdiction of interest, and the sample is a randomly selected group of voters.

Survey sampling is also done in the health area. For example, a survey may be conducted to determine the immunization status of preschool-age children in well-defined communities. Surveys are commonly conducted to determine the incidence and prevalence of certain illnesses. The key point in survey sampling is that the sample be representative of the entire and usually much larger population. It is essential that some random mechanism be used to select the sample in order for the statistical statement to be valid. Statistics are used to determine how close the estimate we obtain from the sample is likely to be to the true, but unknown, population value.

In many cancer nursing studies random samples are not taken; nevertheless, we would like to apply the results obtained from the study group to all similar patients. A typical study would involve a clinical trial comparing two techniques to control nausea and vomiting from chemotherapeutic agents used in the treatment of metastatic colon cancer. A (convenience) sample of patients being cared for at one medical center would be randomized to one treatment or the other. Assuming that study results indicate that one treatment produces a higher response rate than the other, under what circumstances may results be applied to any group of colon cancer patients with similar stages of disease, age, sex, sites of metastasis, and so forth as those studied? Such an inference requires the assumption that there is nothing special about patients cared for at the medical center where the study was conducted that would affect their responses to the treatment. Whether that is true may be questioned in some situations. In studies where it may not be possible to take a random sample of patients, it is important that criteria be clearly stated and that exclusion criteria not produce a highly unusual study group from which the validity of references to a larger group would be questionable.

Normal Distribution

To make inferences about variables of interest, we must know something about how those variables differ from person to person, or time to time. An earlier section included the mean and standard deviation for a set of data. In computing those statistics, sample values are used to estimate the population mean and standard deviation. The actual distribution of the variable characterized by the mean and standard deviation can take on many shapes. The most common of these distributions is the familiar "bell-shaped curve," or Gaussian distribution, or normal distribution (the name used here).

A number of variables have an approximate normal distribution. For example, many clinical laboratory tests have such distributions when applied to healthy individuals; commonly, the errors we make in measurement have a normal distribution. Even when the normal distribution does not exactly characterize the distribution of a particular variable, it may provide a reasonable approximation when the sample size is large and where the actual distribution is symmetrical about its mean.

The normal distribution has some important characteristics. It is symmetrical about its mean; that is, the center of the distribution is at the mean, which is also its median and its mode. If a variable has a normal distribution, approximately 66 percent of the values will be within one standard deviation above and below the mean, and approximately 95 percent of the values will be within two standard deviations of the mean. For example, suppose the diastolic blood pressure for a group of first-year nursing students is normally distributed with a mean of 80 mm Hg and a standard deviation of 5 mm Hg. This is illustrated in the Figure 7-2. By selecting one nursing student at random, we would be approximately 66 percent certain that the student's diastolic blood pressure would be between 75 and 85 mm Hg, and 95 percent sure that it would be between 70 and 90 mm Hg. Looking at it another way, if we continue selecting students at random, only about 5 percent of the time would we select a student with a diastolic blood pressure of less than 70 mm Hg or greater than 90 mm Hg.

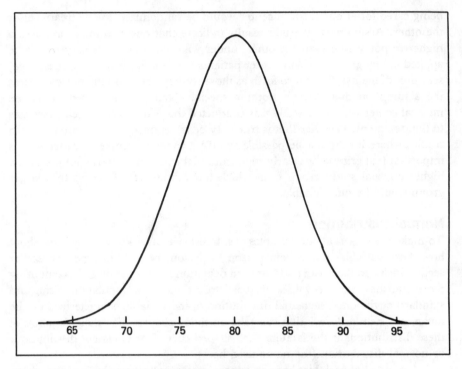

Figure 7-2. Diastolic blood pressure of nursing students.

Central Limit Theorem. One very important fact is that even when a variable does not have a normal distribution in a given sample, in most cases, its mean does have a normal distribution. That is, if we were to take many samples from the population distribution for a variable (all with the same sample size), and for each sample, we computed the mean and plotted a histogram of those sample means, the resulting distribution of means represented by the histogram would be normal. This result is called the central limit theorem. In fact, the distribution of the means has the same mean as each of the samples used, which is in turn the same as the population from which the samples are taken. The standard deviation of the means, however, is smaller than the standard deviation of the population; it is equal to the standard deviations of the population divided by the square root of the sample size (n). In practice, we only take one sample of a particular size, but from the central limit theorem, we know its distribution (normal) and its standard deviation ($S/\sqrt{n}$), which is often called the *standard error of the mean*. Since we are often interested in making inferences about the unknown population mean, we are able to use the information we know about the distribution of the sample mean to make a statement about the likely value of the population mean.

Confidence Intervals. Using the result from the central limit theorem for the distribution of the sample mean, we are able to draw an inference about the unknown population mean. Remember that 95 percent of the values of a variable that has a normal distribution are within two standard deviations of the mean. Since the sample mean, $\overline{X}$, has a normal distribution with standard deviation (standard error of the mean) $S/\sqrt{n}$, we are 95 percent certain that the true, unknown population mean is within two standard errors of the sample mean. We write this as:

$$\overline{X} \pm 2(S/\sqrt{n})$$

and call it a 95 percent confidence interval for the mean. Actually, this is slightly larger than a 95 percent interval; to obtain a 95 percent interval, we should multiply by 1.96 rather than by 2, but it is much easier to remember to multiply by 2. We do not have to use 95 percent confidence intervals; if we want a 90 percent interval; we would multiply the standard error by 1.645; for a 99 percent interval, we would multiply the standard error by 2.576. In reading articles, you may see results reported as:

$$\overline{X} \pm S/\sqrt{n}$$

which, as stated above gives approximately a 66 percent confidence interval. If you wanted an approximate 95 percent confidence interval, you could just multply $S/\sqrt{n}$ by 2. For example, using the nursing students mentioned above, if the mean diastolic blood pressure of 80 mm Hg and standard deviation of 5 mm Hg were obtained on a group of 100 students, the standard error of the mean would be $5/\sqrt{100}$ or 0.5 mm Hg. Thus, we can be 95 percent certain that the mean diastolic blood pressure of the population from which we sampled is in the range 80 ± 2 × 0.5, or 79 to 81 mm Hg.

If we are dealing with relatively small sample sizes, say n less than 30, the standard deviation multiples given by the normal distribution are not appropriate. Instead, the student's t-distribution, also called just t-distribution, is used. This distribution looks somewhat like the normal distribution, but it is more spread out. In fact, there is a different t-distribution for every sample size, and the smaller the sample size, the more spread out the distribution (Figure 7–3). As the sample gets big, the t-distribution becomes indistinguishable from the normal distribution. We must use tables of the t-distribution to obtain the appropriate values by which to multiply the standard error. Tables are constructed so that each line represents a different t-distribution; we must look for appropriate values for the row with $n - 1$ "degrees of freedom," where n is the sample size.

Proportions. When dealing with dichotomous data, proportions rather than means are used to summarize data. For example, in estimating the proportion of patients who develop alopecia subsequent to treatment with 5-FU, we would count the number of patients with alopecia in a sample and divide by the sample size to obtain a population estimate. Clearly, a proportion cannot be smaller than

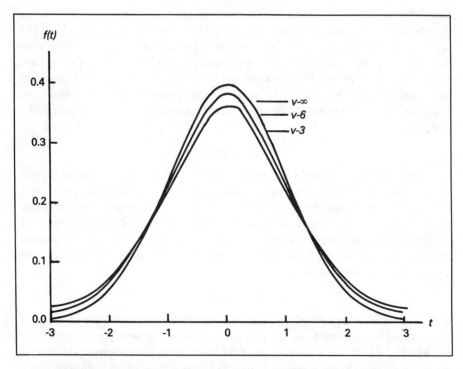

Figure 7-3. Density of the student's t-distribution with three choices of degrees of freedom. *(Reproduced with permission from Afifi, A. A., & Azen, S. P., (1979), Statistical analysis: A computer-oriented approach (2nd ed.), Harcourt, Brace, Jovanovich.)*

zero or larger than one. In many instances, it is possible to apply the central limit theorem to proportions. If p is the sample proportion with the characteristic, and $(1 - p)$ is the sample proportion without the characteristic, and n is the sample size, then if both $n(p)$ and $n(1 - p)$ are bigger than 5, the central limit theorem applies. Thus, p takes the place of $\overline{X}$ and:

$$\sqrt{p(1-p)/n}$$

takes the place of $S/\sqrt{n}$. In other words, the proportion with the characteristic has a normal distribution with mean p and standard deviation:

$$\sqrt{p(1-p)/n}$$

Therefore, confidence intervals for the unknown population proportion can be obtained just as for means. An approximate 95 percent confidence interval for the unknown population proportion is:

$$p \pm 2\sqrt{p(1-p)/n}$$

For small sample sizes, the t-distribution does not apply as it does for means.

When $n(p)$ and $n(1-p)$ are both smaller than 5, it is necessary to use other methods, which will not be discussed here, to obtain confidence intervals.

HYPOTHESIS TESTING

Logical Construct

Often inferences are made in the form: "Treatment A is better than Treatment B." In this case, the hypothesis addresses the relative effectiveness of the two treatments. The logic of hypothesis testing may not always seem to be very logical; nevertheless it is outlined and explained here so as to clarify the inferential process.

The hypothesis is formulated by first specifying a "null" hypothesis in the form: "Treatment A is no different from Treatment B." Next, an "alternate" hypothesis is specified in the form: "Treatment A and Treatment B are different" or "Treatment A is better than Treatment B." (Here the relative merits of the treatments refer to some specified variable of interest.) In fact, either the null hypothesis is true, or the alternate hypothesis is true. A common experimental approach is to take a sample of individuals, randomly assign them to either treatment group, and then see which group does better (if either does). On the basis of that "experiment," the data support either the null or the alternate hypothesis.

Because of sampling variation, it is possible to make a mistake and draw an incorrect conclusion from the data. Figure 7–4 displays the various possible decisions. Note that conclusions are stated in terms of "rejecting" or "not rejecting" the null hypothesis.

The figure shows the two kinds of errors that can be made. Type I error is made when the null hypothesis is true (truth is "there is no difference"), but we reject the null hypothesis (data shows "there is a difference") based on our experiment. Type II error is made when the null hypothesis is not true (truth is "there is a difference") and we fail to reject it based on our experiment (data shows "there is no difference").

| | Truth | |
	Null hypothesis *True*	Null hypothesis *Not true*
Do not reject null hypothesis	Conclusion correct	Type II error
Reject null hypothesis	Type I error	Conclusion correct

Conclusion (label on left axis)

Figure 7–4. Type I and type II errors.

To each of these errors, we assign a probability. The probability of making a type I error is often labeled with the Greek letter α (alpha) and is called the "significance level." The probability of making a type II error is often labeled with the Greek letter β (beta). Often, rather than working with β, we work with $1 - \beta$ which is the probability of correctly rejecting the null hypothesis when it is not true; $1 -$ is called the "power" of the test. Ideally, we would like α and β to be as small as possible. A major use of power is in determining the sample size that we would need in order to detect a "significant difference" (for a particular) of a specified amount between the two treatments.

In practice, rather than rejecting or not rejecting the null hypothesis at a certain significance level, we often record the significance level determined from the data. This value is called the "p-value"; it is the probability of observing a difference as big or bigger than was found in the experiment (or study) of concern if the null hypothesis was actually true. So, by random variability alone, there is a chance we would reject the null hypothesis; this is what the p-value measures. In effect, the p-value is the observed α level. Sometimes it can be computed exactly; otherwise we often say that p is less than a particular value. Commonly accepted cutoff points of α or p that are considered "significant" are 0.05 (or a 1-in-20 chance of erroneously rejecting the null hypothesis) and 0.01 (or a 1-in-100 chance of erroneously rejecting the null hypothesis).

Depending on the types of data collected, whether nominal, ordinal, interval, or ratio, there are different statistical tests used to evaluate the hypothesis of interest. The more common tests that may be encountered are discussed below.

One Sample Test on a Mean

This test is used when data are based on interval or ratio scales. The test determines whether the population mean is equal to some particular value. This technique compares the sample mean to the hypothesized mean. The investigator may do a survey or may actually administer a treatment but does not have a concurrent control. The test assumes that the data come from a population with a normal distribution. This assumption is based on the central limit theorem, which holds that means have a normal distribution when the sample size is not small. The test is reasonably reliable, even when the assumption of normality is not valid.

This test is called the one-sample t-test. The test statistics are as follows:

$$t = \frac{\overline{X} - \mu_0}{S/\sqrt{n}} .$$

Here, $\overline{X}$ is the sample mean, μ_0 is the hypothesized population mean, S is the sample standard deviation, and n is the sample size. We would reject the null hypothesis that the population mean is equal to μ_0 if the test statistic is "large" (either positive or negative). We compare t to a t-distribution with $n - 1$ degrees of freedom. For n larger than 30 we can use the cutoff points for the normal distribution. In either case, if t is bigger than the cutoff point from the table,* we would reject the null hypothesis. Recall, for the normal distribution if $t > 1.96$ or $t < -1.96$, we would reject the null hypothesis at the 0.05 level of significance (ie, the p-value is less than 0.05).

Sometimes, we know that the data do not have a normal distribution and with small samples do not feel comfortable about using a t-test. In many cases the data can be "transformed" so that they are approximately normally distributed. Common transformations of data are to take their logarithm or their square root. That is, sometimes when the variable of interest does not have a normal distribution, its logarithm or square root may have such a distribution.

As an example, consider the following data, which represent survival times in months for a type of myocardial infarction:

$$129, 261, 39, 23, 6, 89, 5, 1, 2, 33$$

These data values are obviously not normally distributed (note especially the largest values, 129 and 261 months). It turns out, however, that the logarithm of the data values do have a normal distribution, and a t-test could be used.

Test for Comparing Two Independent Means

This test is also used with data based on interval or ratio scales. The test compares means from two independent samples, as when comparisons occur between treatment and control groups, each of which is independently selected, or between treatment groups to which patients are randomly assigned. Here, the null hypothesis is that there is no difference in the population means for the two groups being compared. As in the case for the one-sample test on a mean, it is also assumed that the variable of interest has a normal distribution; if the null hypothesis is true, the normal distribution for each of the two groups being compared is identical. An additional assumption is that the variances (and hence the standard deviations) in the two populations are equal. This does not state that the two sample variances must be equal, since they are estimates, which themselves can vary from sample to sample.

The test statistic used also has a t-distribution and looks like this:

$$t = \frac{\overline{X}_1 - \overline{X}_2}{\sqrt{S_p^2(1/n_1 + 1/n_2)}} \; .$$

This t-test has $n_1 + n_2 - 2$ degrees of freedom. Here, $\overline{X}_1$ is the sample mean from one group and $\overline{X}_2$ is the sample mean from the other group, n_1 is the sample size from the first group and n_2 is the sample size from the second group (they need not be equal) and S_p^2 is the weighted variance from the two samples, which is estimating the unknown but common population variance. We compute S_p^2 as follows:

$$S_p^2 = \frac{(n_1 - 1)\, S_1^2 + (n_2 - 1)\, S_2^2}{n_1 + n_2 - 2} \; ,$$

where S_1^2 and S_2^2 are the sample variances from the two groups.

---

*Tables for the t-distribution can be found in most statistics textbooks.

When the assumption that the variances in the population are equal is not a reasonable one, this test is not appropriate. The problem of how best to modify the t-test in such cases has been one that has stumped some of the best statisticians over several decades, and a completely satisfactory solution has not been found. In most situations, the assumption is reasonable. So called "nonparametric" tests are a help in situations when it is not; some will be described below.

Test for Comparing Two Paired Means

As in the previous two tests, this statistic is also used for data based on interval or ratio scales. This test compares two means where the experimental units in the two samples are related. Paired data can occur when a subject serves as his or her own control, as in a before-and-after treatment comparison. This would be a case of "self-pairing." Another type of "natural pairing" can occur when a sibling serves as a control for the subject. "Artificial pairing" takes place when control is matched to the subject on a few characteristics such as age, sex, socioeconomic status, or another parameter.

When this pairing is part of the experimental design, the paired t-test should be used, not the t-test for two independent samples. The test statistic used is as follows:

$$t = \frac{\overline{d}}{S_d/\sqrt{n}} \cdot$$

In this formula $\overline{d}$ is the sample mean of the differences for each pair and S_d is the sample standard deviation of the differences. This statistic has a t-distribution with $n - 1$ degrees of freedom, where n is the number of pairs. For example, suppose we wish to measure the pulse rates of subjects before and after drinking two cups of coffee to see if there is an increase in pulse rate after drinking the coffee. The null hypothesis is that there is no difference. Before-and-after pulse rates would be measured for each subject, the difference would be recorded, the mean and standard deviation of the difference would be computed, then the test statistic would be calculated using the formula given above.

Nonparametric Tests for Comparing Two Means

There is a group of statistical procedures that fall into the category "nonparametric." These procedures make no assumptions or only minor ones about the underlying distribution from which samples are taken. If it is not possible to assume that the underlying distribution of the sample is normal and if we do not care to transform the data to produce a normal distribution, the alternative is to use a nonparametric method to test the hypothesis. Nonparametric procedures are usually easy to use. They are based on the rank order of the data, not the actual values. In other words, we only use the information about the order of the data from smallest to largest or lowest to highest, and so forth. Some information is lost by not using actual values, but not much. Nonparametric tests may be used with ordinal data. Two of the more commonly used methods, analogous to the paired t-test and the two-independent-sample t-test, are discussed below.

Wilcoxon Signed-Rank Test. This test is used analogously to the t-test for comparing two paired means. It tests the null hypothesis that the median of the differences between the pairs is zero against either a one- or two-sided alternative, as appropriate. The procedure requires that we take the difference between the members of each of the pairs and assign ranks to the absolute difference (ie, ignore the signs) between the pairs. Given n pairs, the pair with the smallest absolute difference is assigned a rank of 1, the pair with the second smallest difference is assigned a rank of 2, and so on. If two pairs have equal differences, they are each assigned the average of the next two ranks. Those pairs for which the difference is zero are ignored, and the sample size is reduced by the number of such pairs. After the ranking process is completed, note which of the differences were positive and which were negative in sign. The test statistic is the sum of the ranks of the pairs with positive differences. There are tables for the signed-rank test, which give exact p-values for the appropriate sample size and the value of the test statistic. When the sample size is large, a normal distribution approximation is possible; if T is the test statistic, and n is the number of pairs with nonzero differences, then

$$Z = \frac{T - n(n + 1)/4}{\sqrt{[n(n + 1)(2n + 1)/24]}}$$

has a "standard" normal distribution (ie, with mean equal to 0 and standard deviation equal to 1), and it is possible to compare z to a normal table to obtain the p-value. Note that by taking the differences of a single set of sample values from a hypothesized median m_0, rather than pair differences, the same statistic yields a nonparametric version of the one-sample t-test.

Example. Suppose that the research question asks whether the birth weight of twins is related to their order of birth. We test the null hypothesis that there is no difference in median birth weight between the twin pairs against the alternate that the median of the difference is not zero. A sample of 11 twin pairs yields the data shown in Table 7–1 (weight given in pounds). The tenth pair is dropped from the analysis because there is no difference between the twins; and the average of ranks 4 and 5 are assigned to pairs 9 and 11 since their differences

TABLE 7-1. EXAMPLE OF WILCOXON SIGNED-RANK TEST

Set	1	2	3	4	5	6	7	8	9	10	11
First-born	6.2	4.7	5.9	5.0	7.1	5.3	8.8	7.0	6.3	5.6	7.1
Second-born	6.0	4.2	5.6	5.1	6.3	4.6	7.7	7.6	5.9	5.6	6.7
Sign (1st − 2nd)	+	+	+	−	+	+	+	−	+	tie	+
Absolute value of difference	.2	.5	.3	.1	.8	.7	1.1	.6	.4		.4
Rank	2	6	3	1	9	8	10	7	4.5		4.5

are equal. The test statistic $T = \Sigma$ positive ranks $= 2 + 6 + 3 + 9 + 8 + 10 + 4.5 + 4.5 = 47$. A table for the signed-rank test indicates that 47 is sufficient to reject the null hypothesis (two-sided) at the 0.05 level of significance. Therefore, it is valid to conclude that the median difference in weights between the twins is positive in favor of the firstborn.

The Wilcoxon signed-rank test can also be used to test whether the median of a single sample is greater or less than a hypothesized value μ_0 by substracting μ_0 from each observed value and treating the results in exactly the same way as the differences in pairs described above. The same formula applies.

Wilcoxon Rank-Sum Test. This test is used in place of the t-test for comparing two independent means. It tests the null hypothesis that the distributions from each of the two independent samples of medians are the same, against the alternate hypothesis that the medians are different. The statistic assumes that samples of size n_1 and n_2 are independently selected from two continuous populations. If the null hypothesis is true, the two samples can be combined into one of size $n = n_1 + n_2$, since they should be indistinguishable. To obtain a test statistic, ranks are assigned to each unit of analysis, 1 to the smallest, 2 to the second smallest, up to n for the largest, while keeping track of the sample from which each unit was observed. Tied observations are assigned the average of the rank of the next two observations. The test statistic, T, is the sum of the ranks of the sample with the smaller sample size. If the null hypothesis is not true, we would expect T to be either relatively small or relatively large, depending on the alternate hypothesis. Tables exist to determine p-values but they generally do not go up to very large samples sizes. However, when we have reasonably large sample sizes, then

$$z = \frac{T - [n_1 (n_1 + n_2 + 1)/2]}{\sqrt{n_1 n_2 (n_1 + n_2 + 1)/12}}$$

has a standard normal distribution, and appropriate p-values can be obtained from a table of that distribution.

The rank-sum test does assume that each of the pair groups has the same frequency distribution under the null hypotheses, and hence the standard deviations are the same. It should be noted that an equivalent test that uses a different ranking scheme is the Mann-Whitney test.

Example. Suppose we wish to compare the length of hospital stays of two groups of patients surgically treated for head and neck cancers. We wish to compare the use of an innovative nursing intervention aimed at improved self-care versus standard practice to see if the self-care intervention has an effect on length of hospital stay. Fourteen patients are randomly assigned to one of the two groups, Intervention (I) or Control (C), with the lengths of stay in the hospital (in days) shown in Table 7–2. A Wilcoxon table of T values reveals that the two sided p-value for $T = 24$ is <0.01. Therefore, it is valid to conclude that the self-care intervention is effective in reducing length of hospital stay.

TABLE 7–2. EXAMPLE OF WILCOXON RANK-SUM TEST

Intervention:	35	35	21	33	18	19		
Control:	27	39	37	42	51	39	34	40

Lengths of stay arranged by order:

Days	18	19	21	25	27	33	34	35	37	39	39	40	42	51
Group	I	I	I	I	C	I	C	I	C	C	C	C	C	C
Rank	1	2	3	4	5	6	7	8	9	10.5	10.5	12	13	14

$$T = 1 + 2 + 3 + 4 + 6 + 8 = 24$$

Tests on Proportions

Cancer nursing studies often include categorical data on which it is necessary to make comparisons between two groups as to the proportion positive for some attribute. The situation is analogous to the comparison of two means, except that the comparison is between two proportions. The most familiar way to test the null hypothesis that two proportions are equal against the alternate that they are not is by using the chi-square test. Data are usually organized into a table with the format shown in Table 7–3 where the letters represent the data. To test the null hypothesis that the two populations represented by the samples in Groups 1 and 2 have equal proportions, where the sample proportions are $p_1 = a(a + c)$ and $p_2 = b(b + d)$, we use the following test statistic:

$$X^2 = \frac{\{[|ad-bc| - n/2]^2\}n}{(a + b)(c + d)(a + c)(b + d)},$$

which has a chi-square distribution with one degree of freedom. The null hypothesis is rejected at the 5 percent level if $X^2 \geq 3.84$. The term $|ad-bc|$ means we take the absolute value of the difference (ie, we ignore the sign) and the $n/2$ is a so-called "continuity correction." We recommend using the correction factor; however, some authors do not. This test should not be used unless:

$$\frac{(a + b)(a + c)}{n}, \frac{(c + d)(a + c)}{n}, \frac{(a + b)(b + d)}{n}, \text{ and } \frac{(c + d)(b + d)}{n}$$

are all at least equal to 5. For ns less than 5, Fisher's exact test should be used. This procedure computes an exact p-value. Not discussed here, Fisher's exact test may be found in most nonparametric textbooks.

TABLE 7–3. CHI-SQUARE TABLE

	Group 1	Group 2	Total
With attribute	a	b	a + b
Without attribute	c	d	c + d
Total	a + c	b + d	n = a + b + c + d

Example. Suppose we wish to compare the effectiveness of two antiemetics in preventing vomiting in patients receiving cisplatin. Fifty patients are randomly assigned to one of the two treatments and observed for episodes of vomiting within the 24 hours subsequent to the administration of the drug. The null hypothesis holds that the proportion of patients who do not vomit is the same for each antiemetic, whereas the alternate hypothesis states that there is a difference between them (see Table 7–4). Since the chi-square value is > 3.84, the null hypothesis can be rejected at the 0.05 level of significance. In fact, since the 0.01 cutoff point is 6.64, the null hypothesis could be rejected at the 0.01 level (ie, $p <$ 0.01). It is valid to conclude that antiemetic 1 is more effective than antiemetic 2 in preventing vomiting for patients taking cisplatin.

Analysis of Variance

The previous discussions focused on inferential statistics used with one or two samples given different types of data (eg, categorical or interval). Suppose a study includes more than two independent samples for which we would like to test the null hypothesis that their means are equal. In such a case, a statistical method called the Analysis of Variance (ANOVA) is used. The particular type of ANOVA just described is called a one-way ANOVA. The alternate hypothesis

TABLE 7–4. EXAMPLE OF CHI-SQUARE CALCULATION

	Antiemetic 1	Antiemetic 2	Total
Do not vomit	15	5	20
Vomit	10	20	30
Total	25	25	50

$$P_1 = \frac{15}{25} = 0.6 \text{ and } P_2 = \frac{5}{25} = 0.2$$

$$\frac{(a + b)\,(a + c)}{n} = \frac{20 \times 25}{50} = 10 \quad \frac{(c + d)\,(a + c)}{n} = 15$$

$$\frac{(a + b)\,(b + d)}{n} = 10 \quad \frac{(c + d)\,(b + d)}{n} = 15$$

$$\text{Our test statistic is } x^2 = \frac{\left\{ [|ad - bc| - n/2]^2 \right\} n}{(a + b)\,(c + d)\,(a + c)\,(b + d)}$$

$$= \frac{\left\{ [(15 \times 20 - 5 \times 10) - 50/2]^2 \right\} 50}{(20)\,(30)\,(25)\,(25)}$$

$$= 6.75$$

being tested for the one-way ANOVA is that at least one of the means is different from the others.

The construct of the one-way ANOVA tests is based on dividing the total variability in a set of measurements (based on all samples being compared) into two components. One of these components is called the "within-group variability"; this account for the variability within the samples being compared. The second component is called the "between-group variability"; this accounts for the variability of the means of the individual samples about the overall mean. As a rule, if the between-group variability is large relative to the within-group variability, we would reject the null hypothesis that the means are all equal. The ratio of these two variances forms the test statistic that we call the F statistic. There are tables for the F distribution in most statistics books.

Results from an ANOVA are usually presented in a table. To understand what the entries in such a table are, it is necessary to describe "sums of squares." First is the total sum of squares (SS total); this is equal to the numerator of the sample variance of the total sample, ignoring grouping. SS total is split into two components as described above: the within sum of squares (SS within), which is the sum of the squared deviations of the individual values from the mean of the sample to which they belong; and the between sum of squares (SS between), which is the sum of the squared deviations of the sample means from the overall mean. If k equals the number of samples being compared and n equals the total sample size, the ANOVA table is constructed as shown in Table 7-5.

If we conclude that the null hypothesis of equal means is not true, all we know is that at least one of the means is different from the others. Next, it is necessary to find out where the significant differences are among the means. There are a number of methods for looking at differences, two groups at a time. The simplest is to use t-tests, adjusting the significance level to account for the multiple analyses. Other approaches are Tukey's method, Scheffe's method, and Duncan's multiple range test. These procedures are not discussed here.

ANOVA tests are based on two important assumptions. The first assump-

TABLE 7-5. ANALYSIS OF VARIANCE TABLE

Source of Variation	Sum of Squares	Degrees of Freedom	Mean Square	F
Between groups	SS between	$k-1$	MS between $= \dfrac{SS \text{ between}}{k-1}$	$\dfrac{MS \text{ between}}{MS \text{ within}}$
Within groups	SS within	$n-k$	MS within $= \dfrac{SS \text{ within}}{n-k}$	
Total	SS total	$n-1$		

tion is that sampling is from normal distributions; the second is that the variances in the k samples being compared are equal.

An example of a one-way ANOVA is from a study exploring the effects of discharging patients early after surgery for breast cancer. This early-discharge group was compared to a control group of concurrent patients who were on a normal discharge schedule and a group of past patients retrospectively studied from patient charts. One of the variables of interest was the number of postsurgical days a drain was in place. An ANOVA was performed to determine whether the mean number of days was equal in the three groups. For statistical reasons the square root of the number of days was used as the variable to be analyzed, and the sample was found to be consistent with normal distribution.

The ANOVA table was as follows:

Source of Variation	Sum of Squares	Degrees of Freedom	Mean Square	F
Between	7.509	2	3.75	9.06
Within	99.431	240	0.41	

The calculated F-value is highly significant ($p < 0.001$) so the questions of where the significant differences were was tested using the t-test. The t-tests showed that the means (of the square root of the number of days) differed significantly between the early-discharge group and the concurrent control group (2.59 versus 2.95) and between the retrospective group and the concurrent group (2.47 versus 2.95). The means of the early-discharge group and the retrospective group did not differ from one another. Thus, we can conclude that the concurrent group was the one whose mean was different.

A one-way ANOVA is only the simplest of the ANOVA models. Examples of others include a two-way model in which, for instance, the effectiveness of two treatments is compared in three diagnostic groups. A two-way ANOVA may be used to test a null hypothesis that the treatments are equal, as well as another null hypothesis that the diagnostic groups are equal. Some of the model names you may encounter are: randomized block design, factorial design, Latin square design, and repeated measures design. All of these can be set up in an ANOVA format.

There are also nonparametric analogues to ANOVA. The most frequently encountered test that is equivalent to a one-way ANOVA is called the Kruskal-Wallis test.

Test for Independence
To this point, the chapter has only considered tests of hypotheses on one variable at a time. We will now consider how two (or more) variables may be related to each other. The simplest situation is presented here; in which a sample is classified as to the presence or absence of two characteristics and we wish to determine if those presences or absences are related to one another. The particular test used is a chi-square test. The test statistic and the mechanics of carrying

out the test are the same as for the chi-square test for proportions discussed before. In the present case, a different hypothesis is tested, namely that the two characteristics are independent (or not associated) with one another. Sometimes it may seem hard to distinguish which of the two situations apply because if two variables are independent, the proportions with and without a characteristic will be the same. The key to distinguishing between a test of proportions and a test of independence is the study design. In a test on proportions, we compare *two* independently selected samples; whereas in a test for independence, we have one sample cross-classified as to the presence or absence of two characteristics.

Example. Suppose we are interested in whether there is a higher incidence of nausea and vomiting with cisplatin than with other chemotherapeutic agents. Comparisons could be made between a sample of patients treated with cisplatin and another sample of those on other drugs on the basis of the proportions in each group who experience nausea and vomiting. Alternatively, it would be possible to take one sample of patients on chemotherapy and cross-classify them as to whether they are on cisplatin and whether they experienced nausea and vomiting. In the first case we would test equality of proportions, and in the second case we would test for independence.

The two-way table for the test for independence can be set up as shown in Table 7–6. We know from the multiplication law of probability that if A and B are independent, then where Pr means "the probability that," we have Pr (A present and B present) $= Pr$ (A present) $\times$ Pr (B present) or,

$$\frac{a}{n} = \left(\frac{a + c}{n}\right) \left(\frac{a + b}{n}\right) .$$

If they are not independent, the above equality is not true. So if the null hypothesis is true, the expected value of a is equal to

$$\frac{(a + c) (a + b)}{n}$$

If the observed value is very different from its expected value, we would reject the null hypothesis. (We could similarly find expected values for the other cells in the two-way table.)

TABLE 7–6. TEST FOR INDEPENDENCE TABLE

		Characteristic A		Total
		present	absent	
Characteristic B	present	a	b	$a + b$
	absent	c	d	$c + d$
Total		$a + c$	$b + d$	n

If we relabel the observed values as O and the expected values as E and we sum over all cells, we have the following test statistics:

$$X^2 = \Sigma \left[\frac{(O-E)^2}{E}\right],$$

which has a chi-square distribution with one degree of freedom. In the case of a 2×2 table, all of the four $(O - E)^2$ terms are equal so we can write the test statistic as:

$$X^2 = [(O - E)^2][\Sigma 1/E].$$

If we have a table with more categories than presence an absence, the first formula holds but we would have more degrees of freedom; we determine the number of degrees of freedom by subtracting one from the number of categories of each characteristic and multiplying those two numbers. For the 2×2 case, we subtract one from each and get $1 \times 1 = 1$ degree of freedom. If we have a 4×3 table, we would have $(4 - 1) \times (3 - 1) = 3 \times 2 = 6$ degrees of freedom. In the 2×2 case, it is possible to use the simple formula we saw when studying proportions; it will give the same value as the formula just described.

It should be noted that as this test of independence is formulated, it does not account for any ordering of the categories within a characteristic; it treats them as nominal data. There are methods that can be used to account for ordinal categories, but these are not considered here. It is also very important to remember that the chi-square test for independence only measures association, and we cannot make inferences about causality from such analysis.

Correlation and Regression

Coefficient of Correlation. While the above discussion focused on a chi-square test for independence between two nominal variables, it is often necessary to measure the degree of dependence between two continuous variables. The coefficient of correlation is a measure of that dependence or association (formula given below). Tests of the null hypothesis of independence state that if two continuous variables are independent, their correlation coefficient is equal to zero. If they are perfectly, linearly, positively correlated, their correlation coefficient is $+1$; and if they are perfectly, linearly, negatively correlated, their correlation coefficient is -1. By perfectly, linearly correlated is meant that for every unit change in one variable, there is an exact unit of change in the other variable. If the height and weight of a sample of nurses were plotted on a graph in a "scattergram" and it turned out that these values all fell on a straight line, say for every increase of 1 inch in height, weight increased by 5 pounds, the degree of association between height and weight could be a perfect correlation of $+1$. The phenomenon of random variation makes it unlikely that we would have a correlation of 1; it would most likely be something less than 1, as in Figure 7-5.

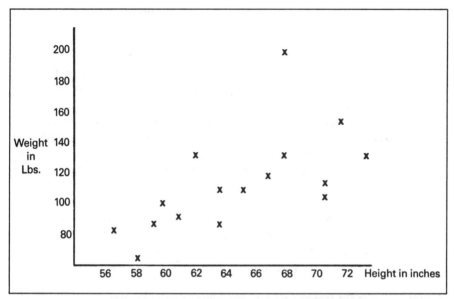

Figure 7-5. Scatter diagram of weight by height.

Interpretation of the meaning of a correlation coefficient can be difficult when it is not zero or $+1$ or -1. As a rule of thumb, correlations from 0 to 0.25 indicate little or no association, 0.25 to 0.50 indicate a fair degree of association, 0.50 to 0.75 indicate a moderate to good degree of association, and above 0.75 indicate a good to excellent degree of association. (Similarly for negative values.) One may be a little suspicious if correlations are "too good," since the occurrence of random variation makes perfect correlations very unlikely. One also has to be careful that there is not some artifact causing a strong relationship. For example, there could be a third variable with which both variables are associated biologically, but there may be no biological association between the two variables being measured. It can also happen that two variables are essentially measuring the same thing, so, of course, they should be highly correlated. It is also possible for two sets of numbers to give a high correlation when they are totally unrelated. A famous example shows a high correlation between the number of stork nests and the birthrate in Northern Europe. As with the chi-square tests for independence, the correlation coefficient measures degree of association and implies nothing about causation.

If x and y are the two variables for which we wish to measure the sample correlation coefficient, and n is the number of pairs of observations, the following formula gives the sample correlation coefficient (r):

$$r = \sum_{i=1}^{n} (x_i - \bar{x})(y_i - \bar{y}) \bigg/ \sqrt{\left[\sum_{i=1}^{n} (x_i - \bar{x})^2\right]\left[\sum_{i=1}^{n} (y_i - \bar{y})^2\right]}$$

This is also known by other names: the product moment correlation, and Pearson's coefficient of correlation.

We can test the hypothesis that the correlation coefficient is equal to some particular value. Most often we test the null hypothesis that it is zero against either a one- or two-sided alternate. Many statistical textbooks have tables of critical values for this test, and all one has to do is compare the computed value r to the tabled value. As n increases, the value of r that gives a significant result decreases. For example, for two-sided tests with 5 percent significance levels, the null hypothesis of zero correlation would be rejected for $n = 10$ if $r \geq 0.632$, for $n = 20$ if $r \geq 0.444$, for $n = 50$ if $r \geq 0.279$, and for $n = 100$ if $r \geq 0.196$. The example shows that if the sample size is large enough, the null hypothesis is rejected even for "weak" correlations. Examples of small but significant correlations can be found in the 1982 paper by Lewis (*see* Appendix).

A nonparametric analogue to this correlation coefficient is based on the correlation between the joint ranks of the two variables of interest; it is called Spearman's rank correlation coefficient. The details of this procedure are not provided here, but the interpretation and the logic are equivalent to that above.

Simple Linear Regression. A methodology that is related to correlation but approaches the problem of examining dependence relationships in a different way falls into the category of linear regression. Here y is considered to be a "dependent" variable and x an "independent" variable when the linear relationship between the two variables is examined. The goal is to obtain an equation of the form $y = \alpha + \beta x$, which describes the relationship. It is necessary to get estimates a and b of α and β. This is done by using the method of least squares. By plotting the points (x_1, y_1) as a scattergram, the least squares line is that line for which the sum of the squared vertical distances from the points to the line is minimum. This method yields the following estimates:

$$b = \sum_{i=1}^{n} (x_i - \bar{x})(y_i - \bar{y}) \Bigg/ \sum_{i=1}^{n} (x_i - \bar{x})^2$$

and

$$a = \bar{y} - b\bar{x}.$$

Once this regression equation is found, several inferences may be made about it. We can test hypotheses about the parameters α and β for which a and b are estimates. We may wish to test whether the slope, which b estimates, is equal to zero, and hence there is no linear relationship between x and y (y would be constant for every value of x). This is equivalent to the correlation coefficient being zero. We may wish to test that the intercept, which a estimates, is equal to some particular value. We can also obtain confidence intervals for the parameters and for the entire line itself. Details for these computations are beyond the scope of this chapter. The line in Figure 7–3 that represents perfect correlation is also an example of a regression line, where $r = 5$. In practice, we would be unlikely to get a slope estimate of exactly 5.

Multiple Regression. Investigators are often interested in the relationship of a dependent variable y to more than one independent variable. For example, we may wish to examine the relationship between the independent variables of duration of surgery, age of the patient, and patient's weight on the length of hospital stay after a modified radical mastectomy. The example includes three independent variables, with the length of hospital stay as the dependent variable. Estimates of α, β_1, β_2, and β_3 would be obtained in the equation:

$$y = \alpha + \beta_1 x_1 + \beta_2 x_2 + \beta_3 x_3.$$

The calculation of estimates in multiple regression is more complicated than in the simple case and requires advanced mathematical methods. However, it is possible to make inferences about the αs and βs as in the simple case with one independent variable. It is also possible to examine the relative importance of each of the independent variables in determining how much of the variability in y can be explained by each of them. The total measure accounting for this variability is called R^2 or the "coefficient of determination"; R^2 can be partitioned to show how much of it can be attributed to each of the independent variables. R^2 ranges from 0 to 1; if it equals 1, the independent variables explain all of the variability in the dependent variable. In the case of simple linear regression, R^2 is just the square of the correlation coefficient between x and y; in the multiple regression case, computation is not that straightforward.

SUMMARY

This chapter presents an overview of statistical principles, logic, and methods. The goal is to familiarize you with these but not necessarily to give you all of the

TABLE 7-7. GUIDELINES FOR USE OF STATISTICAL TECHNIQUES

	Discrete	Continuous	
		Normal	**Non-Normal**
ESTIMATION			
Each sample	Histogram*	mean ± s.d. or confidence interval	median and range
HYPOTHESIS TESTING			
One sample	—	one-sample t-test	signed-rank test
Two-sample paired	—	paired t-test	signed-rank test
Two-sample unpaired	x^2-test	two-sample t-test	rank-sum test
More than two samples	x^2-test	analysis of variance	Kruskal-Wallis test

*Dichotomous data (proportions) are sometimes handled like normal data (see text)

required tools to do sophisticated analyses. That would require a much longer presentation. Statistics play an important role in biomedical nursing research in ensuring good study designs so that the resulting analyses are valid and conclusions are correct. Table 7-7 provides guidelines for when to use the statistical techniques discussed in this chapter.

SUGGESTED READINGS

A list of useful statistical handbooks are provided below.

Cohen J. (1977). *Statistical power analysis for the behavioral sciences.* (Rev. ed.). New York: Academic Press.

Everitt, B.S. (1977). *The analysis of contingency tables.* New York: Wiley.

Hays, W.L. (1981). *Statistics* (3rd ed.). New York: Holt, Rinehart & Winston.

Johnson, R.R. (1976). *Elementary statistics.* (2nd ed.). North Scituate, MA: Duxbury Press.

Keppel, G. (1982). *Design and analysis: A researcher's handbook.* (2nd ed.). Englewood Cliffs, NJ: Prentice-Hall.

Knapp, R.G. (1978). *Basic statistics for nurses.* New York: Wiley.

Mosteller, F., & Rourke, R.E. (1973). *Sturdy statistics: Nonparametric and order statistics.* Menlo Park, CA: Addison-Wesley.

Siegel, S. (1956). *Nonparametric statistics: For the behavioral sciences.* New York: McGraw-Hill.

Tukey, J.W. (1977). *Exploratory data analysis.* Reading, MA: Addison-Wesley.

Volicer, B.J. (1984). *Multivariate statistics for nursing research.* Orlando, FL: Grune & Stratton.

CHAPTER 8

Critique of Research Reports

Marylin J. Dodd

The range of quality in oncology research makes it imperative that the oncology nurse have some competence in reading and evaluating studies published in both clinical and scientific journals, newsletters, and the like. This chapter focuses on a practical approach to critiquing research reports. It describes basic criteria used to judge the value of study findings. The nurse who attains this ability to critique research reports can be more confident about decisions regarding the application of findings to future studies or clinical practice. For more in-depth information on the critique of both qualitative and quantitative research, other references are recommended (Aamodt, 1983; Burns & Grove, 1987; Chinn & Jacobs, 1983; Mercer, 1984; Phillips, 1986).

It is useful to differentiate between a critique and a review. A critique is an evaluation by specific criteria; the focus is on critical appraisal of the strengths, limitations, and general worth of a study rather than a descriptive account. A review is a descriptive account summarizing the major features and characteristics of a study (ie, an abstract of the study [Leininger, 1968]). The difference is that in a critique one *evaluates,* whereas in a review one *summarizes* the study.

An in-depth critique of a research report is warranted when a research manuscript is submitted for publication or for presentation at a research conference. In contrast, the type of critique described in this chapter is less detailed and is meant to serve the reader who is reading published research reports or is listening to reports at conferences. Guidelines for this practical approach to research critique are shown in Table 8–1.

TABLE 8-1. GUIDELINES FOR RESEARCH CRITIQUE

Evaluation Factors	Basic Criteria
General factors	Refereed journal
	Classic in its time
	Author has other publications in area
Conceptual factors	
Problem	Significance stated—extent of problem described
	Severity of problem described
Literature review	Placement of study within previous work
	Citation of essential references
	Identification of study variables
Conceptual framework	Identification of study variables from theory
	Relationship between variables described
Purpose	Definition of what or who is to be studied or described
	Logic flow from previous sections
Methodological factors	
Sample	Subjects
	Population identified, and represented
	Selection criteria described
	Size of sample adequate
Design	Informed consent described
	Appropriate design used
	Threats to validity of design controlled
Variables	Variables described
	Power of independent variable adequate
	Psychometric properties of instruments described
Procedure	Steps of implementation of study described
Results: analysis and findings	Statistical techniques described
	Data fully presented
	Findings logically described
Discussion and conclusions	Findings interpreted
	Findings compared with previous research
	Findings congruent with conceptual framework
	Limitations presented
	Conclusions and generalizations within scope of study

GENERAL FACTORS

Three general factors influence the reader's perception of a research report: The characteristics of the journal in which the report appears; the historical context of the study; and the author's (investigator's) credentials. An understanding of these factors will assist the reader in evaluating the study.

Journal Characteristics

The well-known time lag of the content that appears in books commits the nurse to read journal articles in the areas in which knowledge changes rapidly (Barnard, 1980). It is therefore useful to acquaint oneself with such journal characteristics as primary readership and review process for submitted manuscripts.

Primary Readership. For journals such as *Nursing Research, Research in Nursing and Health,* and *Western Journal of Nursing Research,* the content covers all areas of specialization (eg, maternal–child, administration, oncology, etc.). Historically, the readership of these journals has primarily included nurse educators and researchers. Because of this tendency, articles may focus more on conceptualization of the problem area and methodological issues than on clinical application of the findings. In specialty journals such as *Oncology Nursing Forum, Cancer Nursing,* and *American Journal of Hospice Care,* the reverse is true: the primary emphasis is on clinical application. The readership of these speciality journals tends to be nurses in clinical practice.

Review Process. For most journals in nursing the review process is by referee. Here the submitted manuscript is evaluated, usually by three referees who are experts in the content area or methodology, or both. These referees are "blind" to the author's identity, that is, they neither know the author nor the author's institutional affiliation. The preservation of anonymity between author and reviewer promotes objectivity. The referees, independent of one another, recommend whether the manuscript is to be accepted or rejected. The intent of the refereeing process is to ensure the accuracy and quality of the articles that appear in a journal.

Historical Context

The historical context can be summed in the questions, "What societal and professional issues were being addressed at the time this research was conducted?" and "Would these issues influence current research?" and "How extensive would this influence be?" To answer these questions, one needs to know the dates during which the data were collected. It is often left to the reader to deduce the time period of the study from the recency of the cited references and from the published date the article was *accepted* by the journal. The reader can hold the researcher accountable for addressing major issues that could have influenced the study. Failure to include important issues may be a serious omission on the part of the researcher.

Author's Credentials

In the short biographical note attached to the research report, the author's credentials usually include academic degrees and present position held. If the author is a nurse or is another health-care professional, it is also important to know the author's primary role (educator, researcher, or practitioner). The information is useful in determining the author's perspective and experience and adds to the reader's understanding of the overall study.

Knowledge about the investigator's previous publications can be useful: whether the current research report is part of a program of research (ie, a series of studies in a related area) or one study among others in divergent areas. It can be assumed that if an investigator has been working in a particular area relevant to nursing and has conducted a series of studies, her or his expertise in this area has developed over time. Whereas, a one-time study on a given topic does not connote this same level of expertise, for one study by itself is limited in scope.

CONCEPTUAL FACTORS

The conceptual phase of a research project involves the process of referring to general and abstract ideas from relevant theories, research findings, and clinical practice for the problem area of interest.

Problem

The problem area statement introduces the reader to the research area studied. It provides the parameters of the problem or concept. For example, Lewis's (1982) study demonstrates excellent logical flow of thought from the incidence of cancer to the narrower parameters of control and quality of life. In so doing, she has led the reader from the enormous area of cancer to the specific dimensions (parameters) of experience — personal control and quality of life.

The author or investigator must convince the reader that researching a problem or concept is important to nursing. Research of actual or potential problems in the practice of nursing and their solutions often appears to the reader to be more significant than descriptive studies of the nature of some phenomenon or concept. On whatever level, the reader wants to know how the study contributes to knowledge in nursing. The author must provide this information explicitly.

A clear, complete, simple statement of the specific problem is essential. It should flow logically from the problem area and appear early in the report. It should describe the relationship among two or more variables and imply the possibilities for testing.

Literature Review

The review of literature serves several purposes. It should clearly place the study within the published relevant work in the problem area. The author must describe what previous thinking in the field provides the basis for the study (previous research or reviews). The review of literature provides insights into the investigator's awareness of the range of opinion and findings in the problem area. The research can either replicate a previous study to verify its findings with another sample from the same population or in a different setting, or move into a region of the problem area where there has been no previous research.

For obvious reasons all the literature that was reviewed cannot be cited in published studies, but the reader should learn of the essential works in the problem area (Fleming & Hayter, 1974). The central factors or variables bearing on the problem area should be mentioned so that the reader will not have to guess whether the author was aware of the influence of these variables. In short, the author must convince the reader about his or her knowledge of the problem area.

The Lewis (1982) study is a good example of the synthesis of relevant literature dealing with personal control and quality of life that the reader can place in the context of these variables. When no previous research has been reported in an area, the use of the descriptive–comparative design is appropriate. Lewis included Johnson and Leventhal's (1974) research because it is indirectly related but nevertheless essential and is part of the basis for her study; her review of literature identified the study variables.

The review of literature in the Padilla, Baker, and Dolan (1977) study is inadequate and consists mainly of references. Regarding educational programs, the statement, "unfortunately, these efforts toward change in the nursing care of dying patients have been inadequate," needs substantiation. It is important to explain the statement briefly, since such information would place the study in the context of relevant work.

Conceptual Framework

The need for theory development in nursing has received much attention in the last decade. A theory is a generalized abstract explanation about the interrelationships among phenomena, with the primary purpose of explaining and predicting those phenomena. Theory is the ultimate aim of science in that it transcends the specifics of a particular time, place, and set of individuals and aims to identify regularities in the relationships among variables. When research is performed in the absence of a conceptual or theoretical framework, it is less likely that its findings will be useful in improving our ability to understand or control events, situations, and individuals (Polit & Hungler, 1978). In the problem or concept area of basic science, the theory being studied or tested frequently cannot be tied to an explicit "conceptual framework," but the review of literature can provide a sound foundation for such studies. The need for, and the purpose served by, nursing research that uses a framework is presented in Chapter 4. For the critique criteria discussed here, the reader is made aware of the functions of such a framework.

Broadly defined, a conceptual framework identifies the major research variables of interest and describes the relationship between these variables. The framework should be relevant to the problem area and give the reader an understanding of how it relates to the study. The author needs to describe how the concepts of the framework relate to the problem statement. A framework, whether chosen from nursing theories or from other disciplines, assists in explaining the phenomena under investigation.

Statements that synthesize the literature and framework are often missing in research reports. Authors fail to discuss how pertinent variables from the literature are placed within the framework. Frequently, these sections of a report lack articulation of purpose.

Lewis (1982) identified a conceptual framework by deriving it from the reinforcement paradigm that was an appropriate conceptualization of this area of study. A schema of Lewis's conceptual framework is shown in Figure 8-1.

There are, however, some problems of conceptual flow in the Lewis study. Self-esteem and purpose in life, two concepts that are tested indicators of quality of life, are not explicitly included in the conceptual framework (reinforcement paradigm), but they are subsumed under helplessness. Quality of life, one of the main phenomena investigated by this researcher, is not included as a concept in this framework. It is interesting that helplessness (or the negative aspect of quality of life?) holds a major position in the framework but disappears nearly completely in subsequent pages of the report. Whereas anxiety, low self-esteem, and diminished sense of purpose of life are mentioned as sequelae of helplessness but are never expanded in their positively valued aspects as indicators of quality of life. This occurred because of the low association with control measures and absence of relationship to self-esteem, anxiety, and purpose in life (Lewis, personal communication, May, 1988). The framework does not include any specific bases that would allow future inferences for nursing practice.

Although an investigator has the license to select those aspects of a theory that appear most promising, others may disagree. For example, another investigator might look at social learning theory (SLT) and conclude that the following assumptions are more important than control: (1) In novel or ambiguous situations, general expectancy is more likely to operate; (2) the value of the reinforcement, not locus of control, is more likely to operate when the situation is *not* novel

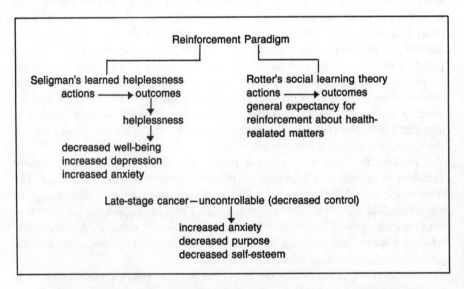

Figure 8-1. Schema of Lewis's conceptual framework. *(From Lewis, F.M., (1982), Experienced personal control and quality of life in late-stage cancer patients,* Nursing Research, 31, *113–119).*

or ambiguous. Because the cancer experience may be familiar as a long-standing illness, the value of the reinforcement may be a more appropriate predictor of behavior than control. However, since the cancer experience may be ambiguous, even though long-standing, as when treatment outcomes prove inconclusive and unsatisfactory, locus of control may be a more appropriate predictor. Thus, the value of providing a clear conceptual framework lies in its usefulness in interpreting study findings to explain the phenomena of interest.

In today's world of exploding information, journals tend to value brevity. For example, in the Padilla, Baker, and Dolan (1977) article, the conceptual framework is briefly summarized in their hypotheses and preceding paragraphs. Death causes anxiety; thus nurses tend to avoid dying patients. In-hospital education programs that teach psychosocial processes involved in dying, and observation, behavior, and communication styles appropriate for dying patients can change nurse behavior. The rationale that supports why such an education program should change behavior is missing.

Purpose

This statement is usually one or two sentences that tell the reader what or who is to be studied. Discussions as to how, when, where, and by whom may be included, depending on how important these questions are to be presented under this heading rather than in the Methods section of the report.

The purpose statement should flow logically from the preceding portion of the report. The reader should be led from the general to the specific. Figure 8–2 depicts this narrowing focus for research studies. The purpose may also be called the specific aims or objectives of a study. In many grant proposals and publications the predictions, hypotheses, or research questions are incorporated into the

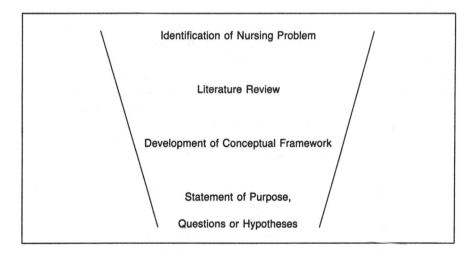

Identification of Nursing Problem

Literature Review

Development of Conceptual Framework

Statement of Purpose,

Questions or Hypotheses

Figure 8–2. Conceptual phase of the research process.

purpose statement. For example, a specific aim may read as follows, "The purpose of this study is to test the hypothesis that. . . ."

Brink and Wood (1978) have derived levels of research. Level 1 is purely descriptive; level 2 is correlative; and level 3 is quasi-experimental or experimental research. For level 1, questions of what, when, where, and who are items that require a descriptive answer. For level 2, "what" questions, like those for level 1, require a more complex answer. The level 2 question requires descriptive answers about the relationship of two or more variables, not descriptions of the variables. Level 3 poses "why" and "if . . . then" or "therefore" questions. Answers to level 3 questions either explain "why" or attempt to establish cause and effect (Brink & Wood, 1978). Both the questions and the statements should include variables that can be measured and are neither too broad nor limited in scope.

In the Padilla, Baker, and Dolan (1977) chapter, the authors pose two hypotheses, an approach appropriate for level 3 research. However, since the review of literature was limited and part of the conceptual framework was incorporated directly in the hypotheses, the hypotheses do not flow logically from preceding information.

METHODOLOGICAL FACTORS

Sample

Discussion of the sample should include information on the type of subjects and how and why they were selected. The sample should be as representative of the population as possible. In evaluating the study, the reader must assess for any bias in the selection of participants. Was randomization used in the selection process? Random sampling requires that every individual within a defined population have an equal and independent chance of being chosen to participate. A table of random numbers is often used to provide the random, unbiased assignment of participants to experimental or control groups. The studies of Dodd (1984a) and Padilla, Baker, and Dolan (1977) (Appendix) use the random assignment technique. There are, however, no guarantees that the experimental group participants are equal in distribution after having been randomly assigned. At best, peculiarities among different participants in the sample are evenly dispersed throughout the experimental groups. Dodd (1984a) tested the four different experimental groups at Time 1 (preintervention interview) and found significant differences on one of the dependent variables. This inequity among the groups was later corrected in the data analysis with the use of analysis of covariance.

The reader must determine if the sample size is large enough (power) for generalization. For additional discussion of power, see Chapter 7. The investigator is confronted with the problem of determining the size of the sample to allow adequate power to answer the research questions or test the hypotheses. In general, the larger the number of participants, the smaller the standard error and the more stable the statistics reported. Ideally, there should be at least ten participants for each major study variable or factor being investigated in a particular study. However, as Fleming and Hayter (1974) note, sample size in itself is not the sole criterion. The problem area determines the extent of the population about which the investigator hopes to generalize. The sample chosen must be representative and selected without bias, whatever the size. The author must provide relevant demographic characteristics of the sample so the reader can evaluate the representativeness of the sample.

In the Lewis (1982) study, the sample size is adequate to test the hypotheses. Some detail is provided for this convenience sample but how the "intermediary" selected potential participants from a pool of patients is not explained. Patient selection criteria are specified and include multiple diagnosis and differences in extent of metastases. But the question remains, were all patients receiving some kind of treatment even if it was palliative? The actual receiving of something might keep hope alive for survival in spite of the odds, whereas receiving nothing might lead to different responses by patients on these study variables.

In the Padilla, Baker, and Dolan (1977) study, the characteristics of the sample are shown in a table. The impact of the nurse education program on cancer patients was tested in ten hospitals. Experimental groups and control groups differed in size at both the pre and post periods. The authors do not explain the reason for the differences, although one would assume the differences to be due to the varying sizes of the experimental and control wards. This raises questions regarding the comparability of groups on all dimensions except the skill of the nurse in caring for dying patients.

If the study involved human participants, the investigator should make clear how their rights were protected. Each participant should have received a complete explanation of the purpose of the research, of the extent of the participants' involvement, and the use to be made of the findings. The assurance of his rights to anonymity, confidentiality, and to withdraw from the study at any time without questions should be presented in the report. The readers should not be left to assume this. This aspect of the report should briefly state the criteria for protection of subjects.

Design

In evaluating a study design, two criteria are important: the appropriateness of the design for the purpose of the study and the validity of the design with regard to the appropriateness of a design. Brink and Wood (1978) note that if little is known about a problem area, a descriptive design (level 1) is appropriate. This level of design answers what, when, where, and who. As more becomes known, a correlational design (level 2) may be more appropriate. This level of design describes relationships of two or more variables. Quasi-experimental and experimental design (level 3) are used when much is known about a problem area and the variables that influence it. This level of design poses "why" and "if . . . then" or "therefore" questions. Therefore, the level of knowledge about a particular problem rather than investigator preference dictates the design to be used. Further information on research designs is found in Chapter 5.

In keeping with Brink's and Wood's (1978) levels of research, perhaps Dodd's (1984a) experimental design was premature, since self-care behaviors of cancer patients in managing the side effects of chemotherapy were incompletely known, whereas chemotherapy knowledge of patients regarding treatment and the effects of intervention on patients' affective state includes more published research.

The description of the design used by Padilla, Baker, and Dolan (1977) for study 3 is not clear. The staff nurses and nurse educators were posttested three times within three months after their educational program. The reader is left to assume that the control group nurses were also followed over the three-month period in a similar manner. Furthermore, when were the patients posttested? Since follow-up of the same patients over a three-month period would be an enormous task, perhaps different patients were used at the posttest. On Table 1, "3 days" appears with no explanation. If this was the pretest–posttest period using the same patients, such testing represents a threat to the internal validity of the design. Obviously patients need to have been exposed to the nurses after the education program, yet who was tested, the same or different patients? When, after three days or three months?

The second design issue is validity. The investigator's efforts to control threats to the internal and external validity of the design need to be evaluated by the reader.

The potential threats to the internal validity of a design include the effects of history, maturation, instrumentation, testing, attrition or mortality, statistical regression, and selection (Campbell & Stanley, 1963). The threat of *history* would be of concern if other events occurred during the study in addition to treatment (independent variable). *Maturation* becomes an issue if changes occur in the participants over time, for example, growth and development of a pediatric sample. *Instrumentation* would be of concern if there were changes in observers or standards for the administration of an instrument over time. A *testing* threat would occur if the effects of taking a test influenced the participants' scores on retesting. *Mortality or attrition* is the loss of participants from study groups. It is to be expected in longitudinal designs; but if mortality occurs unequally across groups, the investigator is obliged to explain this occurrence. *Statistical regression* occurs when groups have been selected on the basis of extreme scores, for example, high and low anxiety scores, and these scores regress toward the mean on retest.

All of the above factors may threaten the internal validity of a longitudinal design more than they would threaten any other design. A one-time design (ie, one data collection) does not afford the same opportunity for the threats of history, maturation, testing, instrumentation, mortality, and statistical regression to occur. However, a *selection* threat can be present in a one-time or a longitudinal study; it results from the biased selection of participants in experimental and control groups (level 3 design) or the sample as a whole (level 1 and 2 designs).

The Padilla, Baker, and Dolan (1977) study reports the possibility of the nurse instructors being biased in their selection of nurses to participate in study 3. The experimental group nurses were better educated and younger. Random assignments failed to disperse these confounded demographic characteristics evenly in the experimental and control groups. A more important problem was the possibility that nurses who were more anxious about interacting with dying patients found themselves in the experimental group. This may account for the consistent finding that nurses in the experimental group were more anxious.

In the Lewis (1982) study, the threats to the *internal validity* of the design involving statistical regression and mortality are not an issue because it is a one-time interview study. History may, however, have influenced the findings during the two-year data collection period. Although the design dictated a one-time interview, the question posed may have elicited different responses from participants interviewed later in the study than from participants interviewed two years earlier because of events either of an internal (maturation) or external (history) nature. Testing may have had an effect since the order of the four instruments was not provided. The reader is left to assume the order of application of the instruments and probably assumes the standard first, second, third, etc. order for all participants. Also, testing late-stage cancer patients with four instruments in one interview may have influenced some patients' responses on the fourth instrument because of fatigue. The number of data collectors involved in the study was not specified. The reader needs to know the mechanism for training the data collectors to ensure uniformity across all administrations of these instruments. As mentioned above, the selection of the participants is not clear because of the confusion about the "intermediary's" role in the process.

In the Padilla, Baker, and Dolan (1977) study, the potential threat of *history* was handled by the use of multiple study sites. This serves as a series of replications of the study. Support for the hypothesis across very different settings provides confidence in the validity of the results despite geographic and environmental differences. The issue of maturation as a threat to the internal validity of this study rests with the nonequivalence of groups in study 3. It was found that the experimental group nurses in some participating institutions were different from the control group nurses on relevant demographic characteristics. This may have led to differential changes in these nurses over time. Again, the replication of the study in multiple sites helps to explain whether maturation had an effect on findings. The report stated that maturation did not account for findings since, despite differences between samples in some institutions, the direction of the difference between groups was the same.

Potential threats to the external validity of a design include reactive effects, interaction effects of selection bias, reactive effects of experimental arrangements, and multiple treatment inferences. The *reactive effects* would be of concern if the Hawthorne effect or investigator bias were evident. That is, the participants are acting in unexpected ways just by being in the study or by reacting to the investigator. The *interaction effect of selection bias* is an issue if the sample has been selected in a biased manner or when because of the treatment (independent variable) some participants or the entire sample are influenced in a differential way. The *reactive effects of experimental arrangements* are caused by the setting or by circumstances peculiar to the particular study. *Multiple treatment inferences* can be a problem when in addition to the treatment (independent variable) tested for efficacy other "treatment-like" events occur to the participants. These unplanned, certainly not designed, independent variables are but one dimension of threat to external validity. Occasionally, investigators plan a combination of treatments to be introduced in the study (eg, Padilla, Baker, and Dolan's educational program). These combination interventions (independent variables) are attractive because of their clinical relevance to practice. They are based on the view that *a, b,* and *c* interventions appear to be helpful to the patients in practice, so why not combine these interventions in one "packet," since the betterment of the patient situation is the real goal of research. The major problem with this view is that the efficacy of *a, b,* or *c* cannot be determined when *a, b,* or *c* are introduced simultaneously. Knowledge of which separate intervention was most helpful or least helpful (or even deleterious) cannot be obtained because multiple interventions are confounded. In the Padilla, Baker, and Dolan (1977) study, the nurses assigned to the experimental group gained in knowledge about dying but not in comfort (skill) in dealing with dying patients. The question of which part of the educational program contributed to increased knowledge and conversely failed to be efficacious for skill cannot be answered.

The report should discuss the threats to the validity of the design and make the reader aware of how these threats were controlled or not controlled and what is their impact on findings and generalizations.

In the Dodd (1984a) study, data collectors were trained to collect data at the postintervention interview. These collectors were blind to the experimental group to which participants had been randomly assigned. Through the procedure of random assignment, the blind condition, and the use of a control group, the potential external validity threats of reactive effects—investigator bias—and interaction effects of selection bias were decreased. In this investigation the sample was also stratified on the basis of referral site, so that subjects were interviewed either in the outpatient clinic or in their homes (Visiting Nurse Association patients). Since there were no significant differences between the participants' responses on the dependent variables, the reactive effects of experimental arrangement (different settings) appear not to have influenced the study findings.

The criteria for critiquing a research report presented above dealt with quantitative (deductive) research. A small but increasing number of investigators are conducting qualitative (inductive) research. Qualitative research seeks detailed descriptions of events, situations, and observed human or animal behavior. In the qualitative approach, the researcher begins with assumptions about a phenomenon under investigation and inserts the assumptions in carefully derived data collection instruments. Examples of qualitative data are: field notes from a participant observer; responses to critical-incident and other open-ended questions. The investigator collects these data without conscious bias.

Aamodt (1983) reports on issues emerging from evaluation of qualitative methodologies that suggest a beginning set of criteria for evaluating this type of research. She states that discovery is the primary motive of qualitative research, and that by the very nature of inductive research, research questions may be unclear, the objectives ambiguous, and the final outcome uncertain in a research proposal, in contrast to the expectations of a quantitative research proposal. Aamodt (1983) identifies the domains of time and space as a major class of assumptions used by qualitative researchers to define the parameters for the investigator's conceptualizations and descriptions. In addition to time and space is the domain of researcher–participant experience, characterizing the activity between the researchers and the participant or object of the study. Aamodt believes the artificial distancing mechanisms of hypotheses and detailed reporting of precise research strategies are neither necessary nor desirable in a well-constructed qualitative design (Aamodt, 1983, p. 399).

Variables

Research variables usually have two types of definitions: a conceptual definition stemming from the review of literature and conceptual framework and an operational definition, often derived from previous research. A conceptual definition is one that describes phenomena in a more abstract or theoretical manner; whereas an operational definition describes phenomena in measurable (quantitative) terms.

In Lewis's 1982 study, the operational definitions of self-esteem, anxiety, and purpose of life are the scores on the self-esteem scale, anxiety scale, and purpose-in-life tests. Experienced personal control was operationally defined as scores on the Wallston and Wallston health locus of control scale (1976) and a one-item question on perceived control over life. These are the common ways of operationally defining psychological variables—scores on tests and questionnaires.

The *independent variable* is that variable that is manipulated or introduced by the investigator. This variable should be described in sufficient detail so the reader has a clear idea of the nature and form of the treatment (intervention). The independent variable is derived from previous research, literature, and theory (ie, from what is already known about the problem area). An intervention is selected that is likely to influence the dependent variables. The power of the selected independent variable must be considered by the investigator and evaluated by the reader. A well-conceived but inadequately powerful independent variable cannot be expected to influence significantly the dependent variables. In the Dodd (1984a) study, the independent variables of drug information and side-effect management techniques were powerful enough to increase significantly the participants' chemotherapy knowledge scores and self-care behaviors, but when combined, these independent variables were not powerful enough to impact on the general affective state of the subjects. The expectation that a one-time information intervention will significantly influence the mood state of a cancer patient seven to nine weeks later underestimates the impact of all the other events the patient experiences.

A *dependent variable* is influenced by the effect of the independent variable (treatment or intervention), at least in theory. In a well-written report, the reader has at this point been informed what variables will be studied. If a new variable surprises the reader, the report has a profound gap in the logical presentation of the study. The dependent variable, once introduced, needs to be defined in measurable terms (operationalized). The investigator needs to seek the instrument most suitable to measure the dependent variable(s). The basic information provided by the investigator about the instrument(s) should include the rationale for selecting the instrument, its previous use (population, setting), detailed description of the format of the instrument; the scoring method for converting responses for quantification, and the reliability and validity data available for the selected instrument.

It is critically important that the research report state the degree of reliability and validity of an instrument. Unfortunately, in most articles, very little information is provided about instrumentation, and the interested reader will have to go directly to the reference for the instrument or write to the investigator.

The primary concern is that of instrument validity, whether or not a tool measures what it purports to measure. There are several types of validity that are frequently used: face, content, criterion-related, and construct validity. An instrument is said to have face validity if, in the subjective judgments of respondents, the items appear to measure the relevant concept or topic of interest. Content validity is concerned with the sampling adequacy of the content area being measured. Experts in the content area may be called upon to analyze the items to see if they represent adequately the hypothetical content universe in the correct proportions. The emphasis of criterion-related validity is on establishing the relationship between the instrument and some other criterion. The instrument is said to be valid if its scores correlate with some criterion. Unlike criterion-related validity, construct validity is more concerned with the underlying attribute than with the scores that the instrument produces. The scores are of interest only insofar as they constitute a valid basis for inferring the degree to which an individual possesses some characteristic (Polit & Hungler, 1978). The instrument is said to have construct validity if scores correlate with other similar concepts and do not correlate with dissimilar concepts.

Reliability of the data collection instruments is of equal concern. If the same participants' responses are repeatedly measured with the same (or comparable) instrument, the results (scores) should be similar or the same. The term *stability* is also used when referring to the reliability of an instrument.

Several methods are commonly used to establish the validity and reliability of data collection instruments. Chapter 6 provides a more extensive discussion of these methods. The Lewis (1982) study provides extensive reliability and validity data on the data collection instruments. However, some additional information would have been useful. For example, the health locus of control developed by Wallston contains 11 items, and Lewis revised this instrument to include a four-point response scale. As with any alteration of an original instrument, it is useful to know why the author chose to do this and how the alteration influences the reliability and validity of the data obtained through the new version of the instrument. The operational definition of experienced personal control over one's life was limited to a single item. The burden of an analysis resting on one item is heavy and unrealistic. Later in this report, Lewis recommends multiple items to account for more of the total variance of this concept.

Procedure

The procedure section of a research report outlines the actual steps taken to implement a study, case by case, from selection and consent to final data collection. Who (investigator or surrogate) did what (independent variable) to whom (participants), where (setting), when (specified in the design), how (form of independent variable), and even why. The why may be implied rather than explicitly stated. Procedural information must be sufficiently detailed for replication to be possible. Another investigator should be able to reproduce the research, reanalyze the data, or arrive at clear, concise conclusions as to the adequacy of the methods and data collection. A detailed procedure on data collection must report how the data were collected (eg, questionnaire, interview, observation) and when it occurred in relation to the introduction of the independent variable (in experimental design).

In the Dodd (1984a) study, complete procedural detail was provided. The investigator conducted all preintervention interviews and presented the information (independent variable) to the four groups of subjects. The settings for the pre- and postintervention interviews were described. Procedural information on the administration of the three data collection instruments (dependent variables) was given. This study could be replicated by another investigator, since the procedural detail is complete.

In Lewis (1982), the author thanks five people for data collection and data entry, but the number of data collectors is not given and there is no discussion of a training session that would have insured uniformity of data collection. In addition, information is required on where patients were interviewed and whether data collectors were present when patients completed the instruments.

RESULTS: ANALYSIS AND FINDINGS

This section should contain a full presentation of the data. The presentation of the data analysis and findings should proceed in a logical manner. If data are omitted, the author should provide an explanation. Every research question or hypothesis should be presented along with the data that will answer the question or test the hypothesis. The statistical techniques used should be described so that the reader can determine whether the analyses were appropriate for the research design, measurement scales, and questions. Significance levels should be reported, and tables should be clear and consistent with the text. Bonus or unanticipated results are reported as found. All interpretive statements are reserved for the discussion section. The reader is referred to Chapter 7 for a more detailed discussion of data analysis.

In the Lewis (1982) study, all data were discussed; results were presented in logical order and related to each of the three hypotheses. The decision as to whether the hypothesis was accepted or not was stated. In addition, the description of the results of the self-esteem, purpose in life (PIL), anxiety, health locus of control (HLC), personal control of life, and control of health scales was stated in the terms described under conceptual framework. Tables were constructed to report the vast amount of data in a concise, easy-to-read format. The data collected on the PIL, anxiety, HLC, and self-esteem scales were parametric data;

whereas the single-item personal control over life datum was nonparametric. Appropriate parametric and nonparametric correlational statistics were used.

In the Lewis study, the sample consisted of a variety of cancer diagnoses, differences in presence, extent, or absence of metastases, and differences in extent of previous treatment for disease. However, the only aspect analyzed was the time span since diagnosis. Statistical techniques could have been used to evaluate the impact of these variables on the major dependent variables, providing information about the phenomena studied.

Because of the lack of description or scoring in Padilla, Baker, and Dolan's (1977) study of the social interaction inventory, multiple affect adjective checklist, and knowledge test, the appropriate use of the one-way ANOVA and t-tests cannot be determined. Similarly, the testing of the hypotheses with the two-way ANOVA cannot be evaluated for correctness. Tables 2, 4, and 5 do show numbers for these measures, but whether or not the scores were normally distributed interval or ratio data remains unanswered.

Investigators who use qualitative methods refuse to claim knowledge of a situation, a linguistic unit of meaning, or a piece of observed behavior until they have gathered enough information to understand the context in which the situation, linguistic unit, or behavior is placed. Qualitative research provides two kinds of data: (1) detailed observation of the meaning of objects and events within a unit of study of interest to a nurse researcher, practitioner, or theorist; and (2) conceptualizations, such as constructs (primitive concepts) that can be useful in building a structure for nursing theory (Aamodt, 1983, p. 400).

As "raw" data are collected in qualitative research, the investigator begins a search for patterns or themes of responses. The reader will note that these themes are not set *a priori* (ie, before data collection begins). The search is essentially for commonalities among individuals, across populations, and for differences across subgroups. The next step is validation of the understanding the thematic exploration provides. The concern is whether the themes inferred are an accurate representation of the participants' perspectives. From this brief explanation of qualitative research, it is clear that the critic cannot use the same evaluation criteria in both qualitative and quantitative research.

In the final analysis of quantitative or qualitative research, the most important consideration is the contribution of the findings of any study to nursing knowledge. The evaluation of this contribution will help place the study in the context of what is already known and what remains to be researched (Fawcett, 1984).

DISCUSSION AND CONCLUSIONS

In the discussion section of the research report, the investigator has the opportunity to interpret findings. The interpretation needs to flow logically from the primary purpose of the study, which should be discussed first, followed by interpretations of secondary findings. Further, the investigator needs to discuss how the findings compare or are consistent with the literature, previous research,

TABLE 8-2. SUMMARY DESCRIPTION AND EVALUATION OF RESEARCH REPORTS*

Reference	Subjects/Design	Variables	Major Findings
Dodd, 1982, 1983	+ 48 chemotherapy patients randomly assigned + to experimental vs. control groups + Longitudinal design	+ Independent variable = written information + Dependent variable = self-care behavior for side effects − Patient recall, poor measure	+ Experimental groups showed significantly greater (<.001) self-care behaviors + Did not wait until effects were as severe or persistent
Dodd, 1984	− 30 radiation therapy patients convenient heterogeneous sample + Longitudinal descriptive design	+ Moderator variables = anxiety and control + Dependent variable = self-care behavior + Patient self-report in log	− Low self-care behavior ± Moderator variable Control significantly correlated with self-care, anxiety did not
Dodd, 1988	+ 30 chemotherapy breast cancer patients convenient homogeneous sample + Longitudinal descriptive design	+ Moderator variable = anxiety and control + Dependent variable = self-care behavior + Patient self-report in log	− Low self-care behavior ± Moderator variable anxiety did significantly correlate with self-care, control did not

Dodd, M. J. (1982). Assessing patient self-care for side effects of cancer chemotherapy. Cancer Nursing, 5, 447–451; Dodd, M. J. (1983). Self-care for side effects of cancer chemotherapy: An assessment of nursing interventions. Cancer Nursing, 6, 63–67; Dodd, M. J. (1984). Patterns of self-care in cancer patients receiving radiation therapy. Oncology Nursing Forum, 10(3), 23–27; Dodd, M. J. (1988). Patterns of Self-Care in Patients with Breast Cancer. Western Journal of Nursing Research 10, 7–24.
*Instructions: When filling out this grid, strengths and weaknesses of the study can be indicated with +s or −s; positive or negative results can also be indicated with +s or −s.

and current theory. Important discrepancies with predicted results or previous findings require an explanation. For example, in Padilla, Baker, and Dolan's study, the second hypothesis was not supported, since nurses who participated in the educational program did not significantly change patients' affective state. The authors explain this lack of significance by stating, "the patient samples may not include any patients cared for by the educational program nurse participants." Further explanation is needed to explain why the procedure did not select for testing those patients cared for by experimental group nurses. Limitations of the study and problems affecting internal or external validity should also be reported in the discussion.

The investigator can interpret beyond the data but should not draw conclusions or identify implications that have little or no relevance to the data. There is no room for statements that have no discernible connection with the research findings. The reader should determine whether the findings and interpretations of findings are indeed those of the report at hand. Generalizations must be confined to the population from which the sample was drawn. This is also true for the presentation of clinical and research implications. One study alone rarely if ever dictates a change in clinical practice.

In the Lewis study (1982), the conclusions were clearly stated. Nonsignificant and negative results were discussed and possible explanations were given including problems with the measurement tools, specifically the health locus of control (HLC) scale. The significant conclusions were referred back to the base theory, making a smooth transition from statistical data to the conceptual framework. Implications for future research were stated, including the need for further defining health as it relates to cancer patients. The inclusion of coping and social support theories into the total framework of this type of study was discussed.

In the Padilla, Baker, and Dolan (1977) study, the authors provide a summary and reiterate the outcomes of their three studies. In one instance, it appears that a conclusion is made ("patients benefited from the nurses' increased knowledge and skill") in the absence of a report of supportive data.

METHOD FOR SUMMARIZING RESEARCH REPORTS

A framework or approach for summarizing a group of studies on a specific topic in terms of critical information, strengths, and weaknesses may be helpful to the reader. One approach is shown in Table 8-2, with examples of how research reports pertaining to self-care behaviors of patients receiving cancer treatment can be described and evaluated in summary fashion.

SUMMARY

This chapter has presented the guidelines for the critique of research. The reader is reminded that one becomes a more skillful and proficient critic with practice. The evaluation of research reports is central to the establishment of nursing science in all arenas of practice. In evaluating research it is important to recognize the strengths as well as the weaknesses of a study to make the most efficient use of past efforts.

REFERENCES

Aamodt, A.M. (1983). Problems in doing nursing research: Developing criteria for evaluating qualitative research. *Western Journal of Nursing Research, 5*(4), 398–401.

Barnard, K.E. (1980). Knowledge for practice: Directions for the future. *Nursing Research, 29,* 208–212.

Brink, P., & Wood, M.J. (1978). *Basic steps in planning nursing research*. North Scituate, MA: Duxbury Press.

Burns, N., & Grove, S.K. (1987). *The practice of nursing research: Conduct, critique and utilization*. Philadelphia: Saunders.

Campbell, D.T., & Stanley, J.C. (1963). *Experimental and quasi-experimental designs for research*. Boston: Houghton-Mifflin.

Chinn, P.L., & Jacobs, M.K. (1983). *Theory and nursing: A systematic approach*. St. Louis: Mosby.

Dodd, M.J. (1982). Assessing patient self-care for side effects of cancer chemotherapy. *Cancer Nursing, 5*, 447–451.

Dodd, M.J. (1983). Self-care for side effects of cancer chemotherapy: An assessment of nursing interventions. *Cancer Nursing, 6*, 63–67.

Dodd, M.J. (1984a). Measuring informational intervention of chemotherapy knowledge and self-care behavior. *Research in Nursing Health, 7*, 43–50.

Dodd, M.J. (1984b). Patterns of self-care in cancer patients receiving radiation therapy. *Oncology Nursing Forum, 10*(3), 23–27.

Dodd, M.J. (1988). Patterns of self-care in patients with breast cancer. *Western Journal of Nursing Research, 10*, 7–24.

Fawcett, J. (1984). Another look at utilization of nursing research. *Image, 16*(2), 59–62.

Fleming, J.W., & Hayter, J. (1974). Reading research reports critically. *Nursing Outlook, 22*(3), 172–175.

Johnson, J.E., & Leventhal, H. (1974). Effects of accurate expectations and behavioral instructions on reactions during a noxious medical examination. *Journal of Personality and Social Psychology, 29*, 710–718.

Leininger, M.M. (1968). The research critique: Nature, function, and art. In M.V. Batey (Ed.), *Communicating nursing research: The research critique* (20–32).:WICHEN.

Lewis, F.M. (1982). Experienced personal control and quality of life in late-stage cancer patients. *Nursing Research, 31*(2), 113–119.

Mercer, R.T. (1984). Nursing research: The bridge to excellence in practice. *Image, 16*(2), 47–51.

Padilla, G.V., Baker, V.E., Dolan, V. (1977). Interacting with dying patients. In M.V. Batey (Ed.), *Communicating nursing research: Vol. 8. Nursing research priorities: Choices or chance* (101–114). Boulder, CO: WICHE.

Phillips, L.R.F. (1986). *A clinician's guide to the critique and utilization of nursing research*. Norwalk, CT: Appleton-Century-Crofts.

Polit, D.F., & Hungler, B.P. (1978). *Nursing research: Principles and methods*. Philadelphia: Lippincott.

Wallston, B.S., & Wallston, K. (1976). Development and validation of the health locus of control (HLC) scale. *Journal of Consulting Clinical Psychologists, 44*, 580–585.

CHAPTER 9

Support for Research

Marcia M. Grant

The purpose of this chapter is to discuss the avenues of support available to the individual investigator conducting cancer nursing research. Support from both nursing colleagues and members from other health-care disciplines such as medicine is critical to initiating a research proposal. Financial support may also be critical to cover the costs of conducting research. Once a study is written, approved, and funded, continued and additional support is needed for successful implementation. This chapter will focus on support before study implementation. The support needed subsequent to implementation will be discussed in Chapter 10.

Although cancer nursing research has some characteristics that make it unique, much of the kind of research support needed and available is not specific to cancer nursing but applies to nursing research in general. When specific cancer-related support is available, it is included in the discussion.

Successful development of nursing research can occur with relatively limited support for some projects. In general, however, research requires support from a variety of sources in order to accomplish problem identification, collection of preliminary data, precise methodological development, institutional cooperation, and cost projection. Nursing support with the investigator's institution is critical and includes administrative commitment and intra- and interdisciplinary support. The need for financial support varies, depending on the nature of the project, but it may be a key element in obtaining the support needed from nursing, administration, and other disciplines. Aspects of support may differ, depending upon whether the researcher is in an educational or a clinical setting.

NURSING SUPPORT

The nursing support available for the conduct of research varies considerably from institution to institution. Historically, educational settings in which faculty achieve high research productivity are distinguished by the following characteristics:

1. Faculty competent in research skills.
2. Research valued as a desirable outcome goal.
3. Role responsibilities include time for faculty to engage in research activity.
4. Compatibility between faculty research activities and the organizational mission and goals (as reflected in the support and rewards for research).
5. Support for and encouragement of faculty's efforts to seek extramural funding for research.
6. Administrative support for research.
7. A psychosocial climate supportive of research and neophyte investigators. (Batey, 1978)

Just how these characteristics are operationalized differs between educational and clinical settings.

Educational Settings

Within educational settings, faculty members' success in conducting research is dependent not only upon the individual faculty member's ability but also upon the philosophy of the school and the nature of the educational program. In large institutions with numerous graduate program offerings, research is generally a requirement for tenure. As increased numbers of faculty in schools and colleges of nursing are doctorally prepared and thus meet the requirements for tenure and promotion, their research track records become important in their status determination. In institutions in which research is required, the faculty member can expect philosophical support for research. If the nursing education program includes a master's program, faculty involved in research are needed to teach research and to advise master's students on theses. If a doctoral program is included, faculty with productive research programs in place are required to maintain the quality of the educational program, give appropriate guidance and support to doctoral students conducting dissertations, and meet the requirements for accreditation of the program. In educational settings in which graduate education is not the major focus, less nursing support for research will be apparent. In fact, educational commitments may be such that only an occasional faculty member is able to carry out research. Faculty interested in conducting research should seek out employment in schools where research is valued and supported.

Organizational patterns of nursing support for research vary among educational settings. The most common approach involves the establishment of an office for research headed by an individual who is a director, associate, or assistant dean (McArt, 1987). Such offices may be funded by the institution or partially or completely by grant money. The responsibilities of such an office consist of assisting faculty members interested in conducting research through research consultation, review of proposals, and assistance with proposal development. Additional services include dissemination of information regarding funding sources, research conferences, and potential publication sources. Some facilities provide consultation regarding methodological approaches and statistical analysis, while others provide secretarial assistance for faculty who are writing proposals for intramural or outside funding and manuscripts for publication. This office is a key link in gaining access to the institutional officials who need to review and sign off grant proposals submitted for outside funding. Procedures for obtaining these signatures are generally found in the research office. The resourceful investigator uses this assistance to the maximum in developing research.

Support services related to implementation of research are provided by some research offices. These services include consultation on statistical analysis, computer programming assistance, computer instruction and analysis. A microcomputer laboratory for entry and analysis of data is frequently provided. Faculty are taught to use these various services, to the end that faculty become more and more self-sufficient as series of studies are completed.

Although organization structures for research support provide concrete services valuable to the beginning or seasoned researcher, the provision of psychosocial support is also valuable. Such support occurs when administration values research and when faculty interact with colleagues who are also researchers. The research values of the educational program are dependent on the individuals who fill faculty and administrative roles. As the percentage of research-trained, doctorally prepared nurses who fill these positions increases, the provision of psychosocial support for new investigators can be expected to increase (McArt, 1987). Because the amount of research support may vary considerably from one institution to another, it behooves potential faculty to ask about these resources and to examine how the institution can assist faculty in building successful research career programs.

Other nursing support needed may be unique to the kind of research being conducted. Laboratory facilities may be needed if the researcher carries out basic science or bench research. Interview or observation rooms may be needed for psychosocial studies. While such facilities are frequently provided and developed for a specific research endeavor, they may be developed using intramural funds, external funds such as biomedical research support funds, or become available as researchers complete their studies or move to other settings (Ozbolt, 1986).

In general, nursing support for investigators in educational settings is growing rapidly in many institutions. This growth is expected to be of great benefit in assisting new and young investigators to develop programs of research.

Clinical Settings

Within clinical settings, different organizational patterns of nursing research support are apparent (Knafl et al, 1987). An initial institutional commitment to research is exemplified by a statement in the clinical nurse job description that specifies that research is a job expectation (Varricchio & Mikos, 1987). Such commitment may be found in institutions with no specific individual or department with a designated nursing research focus. The ability for clinical nurses in these settings to conduct research successfully is more related to the enthusiasm and tenacity of the individual clinical nurse than to any institutional expectation via the job description.

Fortunately, a trend noticeable in health-care institutions in the United States is the creation of a nursing research position or nursing research department (Pranulis & Gortner, 1985). This approach, coupled with the job expectation for research by clinical specialists, has been instrumental in facilitating research in many clinical settings.

The primary focus of research conducted by nurses from a clinical setting tends to differ from that conducted by faculty in educational settings (McArt, 1987). In the clinical setting a larger percentage of investigators plan and conduct valuative research specific to the institution and its problems. Such research may emerge from quality assurance studies. In addition, fewer clinical investigators have internal or external funds for conducting research (McArt, 1987).

Administrative support is an essential step needed for establishment of a viable and productive nursing research program in a clinical center (Marchette, 1985). Such support includes financial support for nursing research positions.

When such positions are developed, the focus of an individual researcher's role is generally either to conduct his or her studies, to conduct a study or project identified by nursing administration, or to facilitate collaborative studies with clinical staff members (Hinshaw & Smeltzer, 1987). If only one position is created, only one of those tasks can usually be accomplished. The establishment of a nursing research department, with institutional support of one and a half (or more) investigators plus secretarial support provides resources to carry out several tasks. With the department model, the researchers are able to carry out individual studies appropriate to their background and training and to the development of knowledge relevant to the clinical setting, in addition to facilitating nursing research throughout the clinical setting (Rizzuto & Mitchell, 1988). This facilitation may include educating staff about the research process, conducting group research, using research findings, acting as mentor to those who can be fairly independent in their research activities, and providing additional support for clinical staff who are unfamiliar with the research processes but have good research ideas and enthusiasm for project development and implementation.

In summary, nursing support for investigators in clinical settings is strongest when a nursing research department is available and functioning. Highly motivated individual nurses may carry out initial studies without such support, provided other aspects of support, such as administrative and peer support, are present.

Educational and Clinical Collaboration

A recent development in the provision of nursing support for clinical nursing investigations is the development of a model of collaboration between academic institutions and clinical settings (Brodish, Tranbarger, & Chamings, 1987; Stone, 1986). Such a model can be useful to investigators employed in either setting.

As the priority for clinically relevant nursing research increases, collaboration between faculty members and nurse clinicians can create highly relevant and feasible collaborative investigations (Engstrom, 1984; Zalar, Welches, & Walker, 1985). Generally, the faculty member brings research expertise via doctoral education and research experience via the doctoral dissertation and subsequent studies, providing the background needed to maintain scientific rigor in collaborative studies. The clinician provides clinically relevant questions, patient access, and the broad clinical background essential to the interpretation of the statistical findings of the study (Oberst, 1985). Together, the faculty member and the clinician can provide the nursing expertise needed to conduct successful investigations. While difficulties in collaboration have been reported (Brown et al, 1984; Felton & McLaughlin, 1976), collaboration appears to be a successful approach used in a variety of settings.

In summary, nursing support provides the critical first step in carrying out clinical nursing studies. This support can be provided in a variety of ways through differing models. It varies considerably from institution to institution. Nurses interested in conducting clinical research would be wise to seek out institutions where nursing support is available and accessible or open to development.

COLLEGIAL AND INTERDISCIPLINARY SUPPORT

Depending on the nature of the study being implemented, the nurse investigator may need support from colleagues as well as members of other disciplines. Examples include staff nurses, physicians, statisticians, dietitians, social workers, and others.

The interaction of nurse investigators with physicians is especially critical for all clinical research. A variety of patterns of interaction with resultant variations in successful research implementation have been described by Kirchoff (1987). Research can be blocked, stalled, and sabotaged. It can also be negotiated, improved, and fostered by positive nurse–physician interactions. The physicians are frequently the gatekeepers to patient accrual. Thus, interactions can provide support for nursing investigations as well as bridge the gap between the disciplines.

Collaboration and support by physicians is particularly evident in cancer nursing clinical studies (Hubbard & Donehower, 1980; Scogna, 1981). In fact, because of the high participation of oncology nurses in medical oncology research, the research expertise of the average oncology nurse may be more advanced than indicated from the academic credentials and more advanced when compared to nurses who specialized in other areas (Grant & Stromborg, 1981; Mayer & Grant, 1987). Such expertise and interest has had a positive impact on the amount and sophistication of research conducted on clinical cancer nursing (Padilla & Grant, 1987).

Other interdisciplinary support may be sought, depending on the nature of the research question and study design. Respiratory therapy, physical therapy, dietetics, pharmacology, and psychology are a few of the disciplines that may be critical in designing a study. While collegial and interdisciplinary support are important in many single studies, it becomes critical in collaborative research. This collaborative approach is likely to increase as a means to enhance research productivity (Stone, 1986). The key to success in both situations is clear, frequent, and effective communication. The implementation of these approaches is discussed further in Chapter 10.

FINANCIAL SUPPORT

Some research can be carried on without any financial support. The single-case-study approach is one method. Another approach involves a team effort, with everyone adding research tasks to their daily job responsibilities (Holmstrom & Burgess, 1982). However, it is not unusual to help with supplies, space, data management, analysis, and secretarial support. When this occurs, several avenues of support are available for the investigator. Sources may vary among educational and clinical settings.

Internal Support

The first source to pursue for financial support is one's own institution (Rimm, 1981). This is especially appropriate if the investigator has limited or no grant-writing experience. In educational institutions, seed money is frequently available through the school or college of nursing, as well as the general institution budget, and is intended for promoting research among the faculty. Funds may also be available from special endowments such as alumni support (Schmitt & Chapman, 1980).

Biomedical support grants from the federal government are awarded to institutions that achieve a certain level of federal funding. They may be found in educational or clinical settings. For example, clinical cancer centers may have biomedical research support money because of the extent of funded clinical research being conducted. Each institution receiving biomedical research support funds establishes criteria by which investigators are eligible to apply for these funds. Proposal requirements for internal funding are generally simple compared to proposals submitted for government funding. Frequently, one to three pages will be sufficient (Gortner, 1980).

Information on internal funds may be found in monthly or weekly newsletters from the administration, in the research office, and by word of mouth. The amount of an award made with internal funds is generally smaller than that requested from either private or government sources. It may not be sufficient to cover the entire cost of a project. However, it is an excellent source for small pilot studies and can be combined with several other small awards to carry out larger projects.

Government Support

Government funds may be obtained from city, state, or federal sources (Gortner, 1982). Federal funds for research support are by far the best established, with clearly written guidelines, standardized submission dates, and an experienced review committee structure. The most important source of information regarding federal funds is a publication entitled *NIH Guide for Grants and Contracts.* Published by the National Institutes of Health, this document is mailed at regular intervals and lists grant programs and deadline dates for grants and contracts administered by the National Institutes of Health. This free publication can be ordered from: NIH Guide, Distribution Center, National Institutes of Health, Room B4B-N-08, Building 31, Bethesda, MD 20892.

Two of the most common methods of funding from the federal government are grants and contracts. Grants are defined as projects in which the investigator develops the idea. While the topic should be one for which the granting agency has a programmatic interest, the investigator develops the idea and the approach. Contracts, in contrast, focus on ideas developed by the funding agency. The agency identifies a particular piece of research to be done, details the work, and publishes a request for proposals (RFP), which outlines the way the study will be conducted and how it will be divided among investigators. Most nursing research funding by the federal government is done through the grant mechanism rather than the contract mechanism. Both methods involve competitive submission of proposals.

Probably the most important federal government source of funding for nursing research is the National Center for Nursing Research (NCNR), which is housed in the National Institutes of Health. The center has as its general mission the conduct, support, and dissemination of information on basic and clinical nursing research, and training. There are available 11 categories of grants and awards related to acute and chronic illness, health promotion, disease prevention, nursing systems, and other special programs. Examples of some of the types of grants are found in Table 9-1. A complete description of the program can be obtained from: The National Center for Nursing Research, NIH, Building 31, Room 5B25, Bethesda, MD 20892. Deadlines for new research applications occur on February 1, June 1, and October 1 of each year. Once submitted, proposals go through a well-established review process, and one of three results occurs: approved and funded, approved and not funded, disapproved. It is not

TABLE 9-1. GRANTS AND AWARDS OF THE NATIONAL CENTER FOR NURSING RESEARCH

Title	Description
Research Project Grants (R01)	Grants of 3–5 years to support discrete projects related to investigators' interests and competence.
Program Project Grants (P01)	Grants of 3–5 years to support broadly based, often multidisciplinary research program with a particular major theme or objective. Can support individual projects within an overall program of research.
National Research Service Award Individual Predoctoral Fellowhip (F31)	Awards for registered nurses enrolled in doctoral programs related to the mission of NCNR. Includes stipend and institutional funds.
Academic Research Awards (R15)	Small-scale research projects for faculty members in educational institutions. Awards may be up to $50,000 direct for 24 months.
First Independent Research Support and Transition Award (R29)	Intended to support first independent investigative award of an individual. Generally for 5 years with total direct costs not exceeding $350,000.
Academic Investigator Award (K07)	For junior faculty members 4–6 years postdoctorate who have demonstrated research potential. Awards include salary up to $40,000, plus up to $20,000 for research costs.
Clinical Investigator Award (K08)	For clinically trained nurses with a doctorate to work under a sponsor at a NIH-supported center program or one of the general clinical research centers funded by NIH. Provisions similar to Academic Investigator Award.

NCNR = National Center for Nuring Research; NIH = National Institutes of Health.

unusual for an investigator of an approved and funded project to wait a year from submission date for actual receipt of funds. The earliest starting date for a proposal submitted for a June 1 review is December 1 of the same year.

Other institutes within the federal structure whose programs of research frequently focus on problems relevant to cancer nursing include the National Cancer Institute, the National Institute of Mental Health, and the National Institute on Aging. Addresses of these are found in Table 9–2.

State funding and city funding mechanisms are similar to those of the federal funding agencies. Information about these funds can be obtained by contacting state or city governments. Turnaround time from date of proposal submission to time of funding (if approved and funded) is shorter than that occurring at the federal level.

Private Support

A major source of financial support for many research projects are private foundations. This mechanism of support is especially appealing today, when federal funds for research are being cut. The most important source of information regarding private funding can be found at most libraries and is entitled *The Foundation Directory* (Gortner, 1982). This is a standard reference that lists all nongovernmental grant-making foundations whose assets exceed $1 million or whose annual grants total $100,000 or more. Over 3000 foundation names, addresses, telephone numbers, current financial data, and names of donors and key officers are provided.

The procedures for submitting proposals to private sources differ from one agency to another. However, one essential difference is that personal contact with someone from the private funding agency is frequently an important, if not essential, asset. The investigator should contact the company and find out what division takes care of funding. Contacting a specific individual from that division and making the effort to talk with that individual about the research over the telephone or in person will be valuable in establishing whether or not there is a match between the proposed research and the private company or foundation.

Private funding for cancer nursing research can be obtained from a variety of sources. Common ones are foundations such as the Oncology Nursing Foundation, corporations such as Abbott Laboratories, professional groups, such as Sigma Theta Tau, and special interest groups, such as the American Cancer Society. Contact information on these foundations is found in Table 9-2.

Proposals submitted to private foundations are frequently less lengthy than those submitted to the government. Regardless of the length, research proposals must be scholarly, clearly written, and accurate. Grantsmanship workshops are offered frequently, and publications on grantsmanship are abundant. These may provide an excellent starting point for the new investigator.

Financial support for nursing research is available from a variety of sources and in varying amounts of money. This support will assist the researcher in covering the costs of supplies, personnel, and consultation needed to carry out thorough and valuable studies.

An additional mechanism available for cancer nursing investigators is the cancer cooperative study group. The National Cancer Institute funds over 20 of these groups. Some groups focus on a specific cancer treatment such as the Radiation Therapy Oncology Group (RTOG). Others, such as the Southwestern Oncology Group (SWOG), focus on multimodal oncology therapy. Nurses are involved in these groups as data collectors or coordinators for medical research protocols. Through the development of research skills in the medical research implementation, official recognition within the groups of nursing contributions has occurred (Scogna, 1981). Nursing committees have formed and are composed of nurses from a variety of participating institutions. Such committees are able to submit nursing protocols for review and implementation by the cooperative group. This participation can provide support for clinical cancer nursing research by way of consultation on study design, subject accrual, data coding, and data analysis (Scogna, 1981). The support mechanism available through these cooperative groups is operationalized in terms of specific tasks rather than the awarding of funds that the investigator uses to buy the services needed for study implementation.

TABLE 9-2. CONTACTS FOR FUNDING SOURCES

Source	Contact Person and Address
Abbott Laboratories Fund	Charles S. Brown, President Abbott Laboratories Fund Abbott Park North Chicago, IL 60064
American Cancer Society	Trish Greene, RN, MS Vice-President for Cancer Nursing American Cancer Society 90 Park Avenue New York, NY 10016 (212) 599-8200
American Nurses' Foundation	Pauline Brimmer, RN, PhD Director, Center for Nursing Research American Nurses' Foundation 2420 Pershing Road Kansas City, MO 64100 (816) 474-5720
National Cancer Institute	Ann Bavier, RN, MN Program Director Community Oncology and Rehabilitation Program Division of Cancer Prevention and Control Blair Building, Room 7A-05 National Cancer Institute Bethesda, MD 20892 (301) 496-8541
National Center for Nursing Research	Ada Sue Hinshaw, RN, PhD Director National Center for Nursing Research Building 38A, B2E17 National Institutes of Health Bethesda, MD 20892 (301) 496-0526
National Institute of Aging	National Institute of Aging Building 31, Room 5C05 National Institutes of Health Bethesda, MD 20892 (301) 496-9374
National Institute of Mental Health	National Institute of Mental Health Room 10-104 Parklawn Building 5600 Fishers Lane Rockville, MD 20857 (301) 443-5944
Oncology Nursing Foundation	Pearl Moore, RN, MN Executive Director Oncology Nursing Foundation 1016 Greentree Road Pittsburgh, PA 15220 (412) 921-7373

(Continued)

Sigma Theta Tau

Sigma Theta Tau International
Honor Society of Nursing
1200 Waterway Boulevard
Indianapolis, IN 46202
(317) 634–8171

SUMMARY

In summary, support for conduct of clinical research and more specifically, for cancer nursing research, includes institutional, collegial, and interdisciplinary support. How much support and how to obtain it varies from institution to institution. The curious and resourceful investigator tracks down the mechanisms unique to the specific institution in which he or she is employed. Collaborative approaches between nurses (eg, instructors and clinical nurse specialists) are on the increase as demands for research occur. Financial support is available from internal and external funds. The external funds are provided by both public and private mechanisms. At the federal level, the National Center for Nursing Research provides support for cancer nursing research as well as other nursing studies. The National Cancer Institute and the American Cancer Society provide support for investigations as well. These support mechanisms are provided primarily for study proposals. Additional support is needed once the proposal is approved. This additional support is discussed in Chapter 10.

REFERENCES

Batey, M. (1978). Researchmanship—nursing research productivity: The University of Washington experience. *Western Journal of Nursing Research, 7*(4), 489–493.

Brodish, M.S., Tranbarger, R.E., Chamings, P.A. (1987). Consider this . . . clinical nursing research: A model for collaboration. *Journal of Nursing Administration, 17*(4) 6–7.

Brown, L.P., Tanis, J., Hollingsworth, A. et al (1984). Conducting research as a group. *Nursing Forum, 21*(4), 174–177.

Engstrom, J.L. (1984). University, agency and collaborative models for nursing research: An overview. *Image, 16*(3), 76–80.

Felton, G., & McLaughlin, F. (1976). The collaborative process in generating a nursing research study. *Nursing Research, 25,* 115–120.

Gortner, S.R. (1980). Researchmanship: A successful proposal for intramural funds. *Western Journal of Nursing Research, 2*(3), 654–659.

Gortner, S.R. (1982). Researchmanship: Research funding sources. *Western Journal of Nursing Research, 4*(2), 248–250.

Grant, M., & Stromborg, M. (1981). Promoting research collaboration: ONS research committee survey. *Oncology Nursing Forum, 8*(2), 48–53.

Hinshaw, A.S., & Smeltzer, C.H. (1987). Research challenges and programs for practice settings. *Journal of Nursing Administration, 17*(7,8), 20–26.

Holmstrom, L.L., & Burgess, A.W. (1982). Low-cost research: A project on a shoestring. *Nursing Research, 31*(2), 123–125.

Hubbard, S., & Donehower, M. (1980). The nurse in a cancer research setting. *Seminars in Oncology, 7*(1), 9.

Kirchoff, K. (1987). Nurses and physicians must interact for valid clinical research. *Research in Nursing & Health, 10,* 149–154.

Knafl, K.A., Hagle, M.E., Bevis, M.E. et al (1987). Clinical nurse researchers: Strategies for success. *Journal of Nursing Administration, 17*(10), 27–31.

Marchette, L. (1985). Developing a productive nursing research program in a clinical institution. *Journal of Nursing Administration, 15*(3), 25–30).

Mayer, D., & Grant, M. (1988). Issues in collaborative cancer nursing research: Identifying and utilizing key research personnel. *Oncology Nursing Forum, 14*(6), 91–93.

McArt, E. (1987). Research facilitation in academic and practice settings. *Journal of Professional Nursing, 3*(2), 84–91.

Oberst, M. (1985). Integrating research and clinical practice roles. *Topics in Clinical Nursing, 7*(2), 45–53.

Ozbolt, J. (1986). Promoting nursing research: The center for nursing research at the University of Michigan. *Western Journal of Nursing Research, 8*(1), 124–127.

Padilla, G.V., & Grant, M. (1987). Cancer nursing research. In S.L. Groenwald (Ed.), *Cancer nursing: Principles and practice* (827–853). Boston: Jones & Barlett.

Parnulis, M., & Gortner, S. (1985). Researchmanship: Characteristics of productive research environments in nursing. *Western Journal of Nursing Research, 7*(1), 127–131.

Rimm, E.A. (1981). Funding for nursing research. *AORN Journal, 34*(1), 56–62.

Rizzuto, C., & Mitchell, M. (1988). Research in service settings. *Journal of Nursing Administration, 18*(2), 32–35.

Schmitt, M.H., & Chapman, M.K. (1980). Alumni involvement in nursing research development. *Nursing Outlook, 28*(9), 572–574.

Scogna, D.M. (1981). Nursing research in a cancer cooperative group setting. *Cancer Nursing, 4*(4), 277–280.

Stone, K.S. (1986). Collaborative research: The future." *CNR Voice: College of Nursing, The Ohio State University, 36,* 1.

Varricchio, C., & Mikos, D. (1987). Research: Determining feasibility in a clinical setting. *Oncology Nursing Forum, 14*(1), 89–90.

Zalar, M., Welches, L.J., Walker, D.D. (1985). Nursing consortium approaches to increase research in service settings. *Journal of Nursing Administration, 15*(7,8), 36–41.

CHAPTER 10

Strategies for Project Implementation

Paula Anderson

The purpose of this chapter is to summarize the principal components of successful management of a research project: satisfactory coordination of the research team, efficient collection of data, and accurate management of the budget.

THE RESEARCH TEAM

The research team is the critical ingredient that is primarily responsible for the success or failure of a project. The team may consist of one or more of each of the following: principal investigators, coinvestigators, biostatisticians, project directors, research assistants, data managers, secretaries, and consultants. The complexity of the team is determined largely by the number, diversity, and autonomy of its members and participating institutions.

Cooperative or Collaborative Groups

A typical example of a very complex team that is familiar to many cancer nurses is a cooperative group such as the Radiation Therapy Oncology Group (RTOG). RTOG research protocols have a principal investigator and coinvestigators, as well as a biostatistical core that handles the randomization schedule, data management, and analysis for the overall project. However, each participating institution also has its own principal investigator responsible for the conduct of the study at that agency as well as its own data managers responsible for accruing subjects, collecting data, and preparing the coding sheets to be sent to the biostatistical core. This type of research team is usually labeled a cooperative *group* or collaborative *group* to emphasize the level of autonomy that exists among the members of the *research group*. Although most protocols that emerge from cooperative groups are medical, a few focus on nursing problems.

Some outstanding collaborative groups have emerged in nursing and have been described to provide guidelines for others who would engage in this type of research structure (Bergstrom et al, 1984; Lancaster, 1985). One author (Lancaster, 1985) discusses the six Cs of collaborative research as "contribution, communication, commitment, consensus, compatibility, and credit." By its very nature, collaborative research requires an attitude of sharing of self and expertise. Collaborators are viewed as functioning on peer levels, each member contributing equal and necessary portions. Collaborators may have one member in charge of budget, one act as tie breaker to avoid an impasse in decision making, one act as project director, and all may be responsible for data collection. The collaborative group is the least common type of nursing research team, but it has been established as an important team structure for projects that require a broad base of subjects and expertise.

One-Leader Research Team

In contrast to the peer-member collaborative group, the more common research team structure is organized around one well-defined leader from one institution, and the team operates with clear lines of authority and responsibility. The remainder of the chapter will focus on this type of research team.

Investigators and Consultants. During the planning and approval phases of a project, the investigators and consultants with their varied areas of expertise and community contacts take center stage. Their professional contacts and liaison role in the facilities they represent increase the team's power to negotiate for institutional approval, as well as its access to potential subjects. Consultants provide balance to the team through their particular areas of expertise, be it statistical analysis, nursing theory, dietetics, or other pertinent disciplines.

The principal investigator exercises final authority over all aspects of the research plan and is ultimately responsible for the scientific merit of the study, for the protection of subjects, for the accuracy of the data collected, and for the interpretation of results. The principal investigator's professional integrity determines the overall merit of the project, while the principal investigator's ability to maintain control over the direction of the project influences the degree to which the final product matches the original proposal. The principal investigator may carry out all aspects of a project, as is the case with master's theses or doctoral dissertations.

Project Director. Large projects with sufficient funding may include a project director. A job description for project directors is provided in Table 10–1. The project director reports directly to the principal investigator. It is

TABLE 10-1. NURSING PROJECT DIRECTOR

Definition: The nursing project director is a registered professional nurse with a current state nursing license who is responsible to the director of nursing research or to the principal investigator of a grant under which the research assistant II is hired and assists in the conduct of nursing research studies or activities.*

Qualifications:
1. Current registered nurse license.
2. At least a bachelor of science in nursing, master's degree preferred.
3. At least 3 years of clinical experience in nursing and two of research experience.
4. Demonstrated behavior reflecting understanding of research procedural requirements, reliability in carrying out assignments, commitment to assignments, and ability to work within the framework of a hospital and a nursing organization.

Responsibilities:
1. Assists in meeting the purpose and objectives of the research project by fulfilling a wide variety of research assignments related to the department program of studies and other activities.
2. Establishes familiarity with hospital organization and lines of communication, so as to be able to carry out research assignments in the clinical setting.
3. Acts as project coordinator (implementing a project and managing the budget).
   a. Develops, pilot tests, and revises various research tools to be used in data collection.
   b. Coordinates liaison activities between funded faculty and all outside agencies.
   c. Develops system of tracking potential subjects at each facility.
   d. Establishes data dictionary system to record all supplemental project information.
   e. Reviews all incoming data and checks all coding for accuracy.
   f. Maintains easy retreival system for filing patient data.
   g. Communicates frequently with principal investigator regarding the project.
   h. Participates in establishing a system of computer data entry for the project data.
   i. Works with principal investigator to monitor budget expenses.
4. Trains and directs research assistants.
   a. Supervises all research assistants on a daily basis and coordinates data collection.
   b. Monitors reliability of research assistant's data at frequent intervals.
   c. Collects research data when research assistant is unavailable.
5. Promotes professional self-development.

*All research and experimentation on human subjects is conducted in accordance with the Medical Center's Code of Ethics based on the principles cited in the Declaration of Helsinki of June 1964 and the American Nurses' Association Guidelines and DHEW Policy on Protection of Human Subjects.

important for the project director to commit to the project for the entire period. The project director is the key person in the organizing and daily working of the project. It is essential that the project director thoroughly understand the study, possess an ability to organize each detail of the study, communicate effectively with all levels of the team, be proficient and current in the subject matter studied, and maintain a sense of humor (Rettig, 1980).

In addition, without the support of a good secretarial staff the project will take forever to begin and end (Table 10–2).

Research Assistants. During the data collection phase of the project, the research assistants are the most irreplaceable members of the group. To promote efficiency, research assistants report directly to the project director. The project director reports to the principal investigator, who is ultimately responsible for the project. It is imperative that research assistants match project requirements and fit in with the research team. The fact that research projects are typically pressured by time precludes the luxury of hiring mistakes. Therefore, it is helpful

TABLE 10–2. SECRETARY

Definition: The research secretary I performs various secretarial and clerical duties in assisting the director of nursing research and education to carry out departmental responsibilities and operations. The secretary is responsible to the director and to other members of the department with approval of the director.

Qualifications: This person must be a high school graduate with the following technical skills: typing, above-average spelling, legible handwriting, ability to organize work and meet realistic work load. Minimum of one year's experience performing secretarial duties required. Knowledge of word processing or computers desired. Personality and appearance must be acceptable for a receptionist. A sincere interest in self-development within this role is required.

Responsibilities: This person's responsibilities are as follows:
1. Receives telephone calls and screens, transferring messages or relaying calls as necessary, necessitating a knowledge of the whereabouts of members of the department staff and current general information relating to the department.
2. Performs a variety of general typing duties such as general correspondence, course outlines, lesson plans, instructional materials, departmental forms, calendar of events. Occasionally types from taped dictation.
3. Operates a word processor for typing of manuscripts, papers, course outlines, etc.
4. Operates copying machines for copying articles, manuscripts, papers, student and instructor booklets for courses, etc. Gets journals from library and photocopies articles.
5. Files and catalogues research articles and books.
6. Provides vacation coverage for department secretary. (This person will be cross-trained).
7. Performs other duties as necessary and directed.

Physical Demands: Tactful, pleasant and cooperative attitude, neat appearance. Able to organize work load despite frequent interruptions. Able to do accurate, neat work; work under occasional pressure, readjust priorities. Able to keep information confidential. Able to sit for long periods and walk to other buildings to pick up supplies, stand for long periods at copying machines, deliver materials.

for the project director, together with the principal investigator, to identify the essential professional qualifications and desired personality characteristics needed in the research assistants before interviewing begins. The interviewing and subsequent elimination of candidates then becomes a more structured process. Table 10–3 provides a list of interview questions that have proved useful when hiring research assistants.

In our experience, several characteristics important for research assistants have surfaced. A high energy level and consistent self-motivation are needed. This may be indicated by the energy invested in the interview, professional or personal achievement, or current involvements. It is much easier for a project director to lead high-energy people than to try and breathe life into a lazy buzzard. It is also important for the interviewers to determine if the candidate is overcommitted in the energy department and has sufficient emotional space to feel ownership for the project. During the interview, if there is interest in the candidate, it is important to stress the need for a minimum commitment of one year to the study. It is very costly in time, money, and lost subjects to reorient new personnel in the middle of any project.

The ideal research assistant must thrive on independent work and yet be willing to report in daily. The study may require extensive travel between

TABLE 10–3. SCREENING QUESTIONS FOR INTERVIEWING RESEARCH ASSISTANT CANDIDATES

In addition to the standard preemployment interview questions, these may be helpful in identifying a potential data collector:
   Describe your current nursing practice.
   Describe your experience with oncology patients.

Are you comfortable with patients who may have facial protheses, colostomies, or open wounds (whatever applies to your patient population)?

How would you rate your communication skills?
Are you comfortable speaking to groups?
How do you usually cope with resistance from staff?

To assess the ability to work within a variety of institutions:
   Are you able to function within an existing framework without feeling the need to change it?
   What is the amount of detailed work in your present job?
   How do you usually cope with numbers?

Ability to be objective:
   Do you think you can assess a patient without intervening as you have been trained to do?

Motivation to obtain subjects:
   Are you a person who takes the initiative?
   When institutional liaison breaks down, how would you attempt to build it back? Obtain subjects?

participating agencies for data collection, as well as extended periods without direct supervision. Asking for examples of independent decision making in the applicant's past employment is helpful. Although independence is necessary, in one very large study with data collection in three counties, we tried to provide long-distance supervision and consultation by arranging for either the project director or principal investigator to be available to the research assistants by telephone.

Another desirable characteristic in a research assistant is accuracy in coding and compulsiveness in seeking every possible subject and following through with each subject. Compulsiveness and accuracy may be natural personality traits or learned behaviors; whatever the genesis, they will contribute to the success of the study.

Research assistants must also have fine social skills, since they will be approaching subjects to obtain consent and interacting with personnel in one or more data collection sites. A certain amount of clinical sensitivity is important because patients may be in various stages of illness. In one study about patients with colon cancer (Padilla & Grant, 1982), a preterminal patient asked to be a study subject and also to be photographed as part of a teaching component. Though the research assistant had to allow the patient to participate, it was essential to do so with the utmost in tact and graciousness because the patient was dying.

Often a candidate will possess some, but not all, of the desired characteristics or professional qualifications. The research team "fit" often is more important than many other factors. The "team fit" concept is especially important when more than one research assistant is collecting data. Hiring people with comparable energy levels, qualifications, and skills can help to prevent any superiority feelings on peer levels. There is a tightrope to be walked between fostering a bit of healthy competition that generates project energy and allowing the competition to breed dissent. The project director must be constantly aware of balance in assignments, morale, fatigue levels, and subtle messages. The project director is always in the role of protecting the integrity of the study, and this means daily contact with the research assistants regarding anything that may affect the project. A job description for research assistants is found in Table 10–4.

Orientation Period. Since it is very difficult to hire experienced research assistants, the orientation and training period are critical. During this time, the commitment of the principal investigator and project director to the study and their scientific values should become obvious. It is to be hoped that these attitudes will be absorbed by the research assistants. This is a time for the assistants to develop ownership of the project and to begin to understand the specific aims of the study. The length of the orientation is dependent upon the complexity of the study and the data collection tools. It may range from one or two days for a simple project to 2 months for a very complex study.

At the beginning of the orientation period, the project director and research assistants are given copies of the research proposal to review. As the orientation progresses, each "tries out" all the data collection tools to determine what revi-

TABLE 10-4. NURSING RESEARCH ASSISTANT

Definition: The nursing research assistant is a registered professional nurse with a current California license who is responsible to the director of nursing research or to the principal investigator of a grant under which the research assistant is hired and assists in the conduct of nursing research studies and activities.*

Qualifications:
1. Graduation from an accredited school of nursing with current registered nurse's license.
2. Bachelor of science in nursing preferred.
3. At least 3 years of recent (within past 3 years) clinical experience in nursing and some recent (within past 3 years) research experience.
4. Demonstrated behavior reflecting understanding of research procedural requirements, reliability in carrying out assignments, commitment to assignments, and ability to work within the framework of a hospital and a nursing organization. Experience in supervision and instruction preferred.

Responsibilities:
1. Assists in meeting the purpose and objectives of the Nursing Research Department by fulfilling a wide variety of research assignments related to the department program of studies and other activities.
2. Establishes familiarity with hospital organization and lines of communication so as to be able to carry out research assignments in the clinical setting.
3. Establishes liaison with each facility as assigned and interacts as needed with the investigators, supervisors, head nurses, and medical and nursing staff in order to establish an effective working relationship.
4. Establishes a mechanism to locate all patients who are candidates for the study.
5. Obtains verbal and written patient consent for participation in the study.
6. Provides for the orientation of all agency staff to the project as is necessary.
7. Collects study data in the hospital as outlined in the research project.
8. Codes all study data from the patient and the chart.
9. Maintains communication lines with the project director and principal investigators as to institutional status, data collection, and subject response.
10. Records all mileage and expenses incurred in the course of data collection for reimbursement.
11. Maintains accurate records of patient participation in the study and any unusual events observed in each facility.
12. Trains and directs other research assistants when assigned such responsibility.
13. Promotes professional self-development.
14. Assists with other components of the project as is necessary.

*All research and experimentation on human subjects is conducted in accordance with the Medical Center's Code of Ethics, based on the principles cited in the Declaration of Helsinki of June 1964 and the American Nurses' Association Guidelines and DHEW Policy on Protection of Human Subjects.

sions are needed. Commitment, interest, ownership, and understanding are developed during tool revision and pilot testing. The project director and research assistants practice on each other. This practice includes obtaining a consent, collecting data with every tool, and responding to anticipated questions by nursing and medical staff, and dealing with patient or family concerns. Both videotaping and role-playing approaches teach the research staff to fine-tune the data collection methods. The research assistants watch each other practice but do not critique each other during the training period. The project director maintains that responsibility in order to create a receptive atmosphere and to clearly delineate authority. The goal of the training period is for all research assistants to collect data and code in the same reliable manner. Practice is continued until there is a 90 to 95 percent intra- and interrater agreement with each other, the project director, or principal investigator. Inevitably, one research assistant will achieve this before the others. That individual is then used as a model to help the others.

DATA COLLECTION

Rater Reliability

Reliability checks are made every 1 to 2 months on each tool. To do this, the project director accompanies each research assistant when she or he sees a patient. The research assistant introduces the project director as someone who is learning about the project, rather than as a supervisor. The project director sits out of the patient's direct view and silently codes along with the research assistant, never interrupting the interview. The project director's role is not announced to the subject because patients seem to have a need to "protect" the research assistants by expounding on their many virtues, thus embarrassing the research assistant and distracting everyone from the task at hand.

Data Collection Sites

At each data collection site, time is spent discussing the most efficient resources for finding potential subjects. These sources may include census reports, new registration sheets, the clinical specialist, head nurse, or nursing clerk. Once the best method is discovered, the research assistants are trained to take on the full responsibility for subject accrual. They are repeatedly reminded in the early stages of the study to take total initiative for subject accrual at the facilities assigned to them. The participating institutional nursing staff is not expected to be responsible for identifying possible subjects. In our experience, it takes a long time and a great deal of repetition for research assistants to understand their role in subject accrual.

Role Conflict: Clinician versus Researcher

Nurse research assistants experience internal conflict between their previous role as a nursing-care provider and their present role of data collector (Kaempfer, 1982; McHugh & Johnson, 1980). As nurses they have been trained and educated to solve patient problems by assessment and direct intervention. Hours are spent helping the nurse research assistants to rethink and redirect their energies to nonintervention in order not to influence the study data. However, when patient safety is in jeopardy, the research assistants are expected to intervene as is necessary and appropriate.

If a research assistant does intervene, this action needs to be reported to the project director. Because of the severity of disease of some study subjects and the high potential for research assistant intervention, some data collection tools may need a data entry column to indicate when actual intervention has been necessary.

It is also necessary to teach the patient subjects about the nurse research assistant role. Patients are accustomed to seeing a nurse function in a certain manner and often try to use the research assistant as a private duty nurse or as a means of obtaining a staff nurse. A standard response taught the research assistants is, "We are guests in this hospital and unfamiliar with the routine. It would be better if you would put on your call light. . . ." This response helps research staff avoid being caught in the middle between the patient and staff. It is important to be cautious about stepping beyond the limits of the study. The research assistants are expected to collect data, not impact on them through their interventions.

Translations

Occasionally there are enough potential subjects that do not speak English to warrant having all data collection tools translated. These translations should be evaluated for reliability and validity. An interpreter can be used to help obtain a consent and administer questionnaires that are written in the native language. When an interpreter is used, that individual should participate in a minitraining program to make sure she or he is functioning on the project in precisely the same way as the research assistant.

Tool Format

At the same time the research assistants are in training, the project director, under the supervision of the principal investigator and biostatistician, should be setting up each tool for computerization of data. Each questionnaire must include a subject number on every page in case the pages become separated, the correct number of data entry fields (formerly called key-punch columns for those who still remember using 80-column key-punch cards) for each variable, and if the questionnaire is administered more than once, a time-given field. For studies involving several facilities, a code for each agency is essential. Tools should be designed consistently with subject number, time given, and facility appearing in order in the same place (eg, upper right corner) of every instrument. Studies involving a number of facilities or patient units may assign specific nurse and patient subject numbers to minimize error.

Project Manuals

Research Assistant's Manual. A loose-leaf notebook is recommended to organize and standardize the data management procedure for research assistants. It is divided into two major sections: Data Collection and Data Dictionary. The sections are tabbed for easy location of desired information.

The data collection section may include information on how to obtain a consent, standard information that is given to potential subjects about the study, standard staff orientation content for each facility, and details about each agency such as parking, location, and expenses, nurses' names and extension numbers, locations of medical records, cafeteria, and anything else that may be helpful (Table 10–5). The data dictionary section may include a tab for each data-collection tool, rules for coding for each tool, and subject listing. The notebook sections are identical for all research assistants and make data collection and coding a much easier task. All tool corrections and supplemental coding information are written directly into the manual in the appropriate section. For instance if the question is whether the patient has had chemotherapy and if so, what type, each course of chemotherapy is assigned a code number, and these code numbers are recorded for later reference on the tool. As the study progresses, there may be 50 different chemotherapy combinations. If the chemotherapy does not appear in the dictionary, the research assistant assigns it the next appropriate number and then circulates the information to all research assistants and the project director so they may add it to their data dictionaries. Thus, every notebook is identical and up-to-date. We have found this method *very* efficient.

Project Director's Manual. The project director's notebook varies somewhat in that there is a section for subjects accrued. In this section each subject is listed, with space to record the date when each research tool was completed (Table 10–6). It is a quick reference for the amount of data that has been retrieved and serves as a place to keep track of missing data, withdrawals from the study, and any other important patient specific information.

Analysis Manual. The analysis manual includes pertinent information about the sample and results. Each analysis (usually resulting in a computer printout) is

---

TABLE 10-5. SECTIONS OF RESEARCH ASSISTANT MANUAL*

Data Collection Information
    Format of orientation to facilities
    Consent forms and guidelines for use (how many copies and placement)
    Presentation of project to potential subject
    Standardized responses of commonly asked questions about the study
    Pre- and posttests with keys if applicable
    Diary of any changes that apply to this section
    Facility information

Data Dictionary Information
    Time-line sheet indicating week by week the data to be collected
    Listing of all tools, time-given code, and key-punch card numbers if applicable
    Instructions for coding each tool
    Copy of all tool revisions with date
    Coding additions
    Listing by subject name and number the dates of all data collected or missing (project director's notebook only)

*Each section is tabbed for easy location.

TABLE 10-6. TRACKING SYSTEMS OF SUBJECTS AND INSTRUMENTS

Time Period	Tools	Subjects	001	002	003
First Observation (pretreatment)	Locus of control Health states				
Second Observation (during treatment)	Quality of life Daily care of side effects				
Third Observation (end of treatment)	Oral assessment Satisfaction with care providers				

given a number code. Tables, charts, and graphs summarizing the analyses are filed in the analysis manual with the same number code as the computer printout from whence they were derived. After these summary tables have been checked for accuracy, they are initialed by the principal investigator. In this manner, all coinvestigators have an organized method by which to refer to the computer printouts and tables for subsequent preparation of scientific articles and presentations.

Institutional Cooperation

Medical and nursing staff are the gatekeepers. They protect patient subjects (Cronenwett, 1986). A collegial relationship established with the hospital and nursing administration of potential facilities will ease the entrée into the institutions (Flaskerud & Janken, 1978). Physician approval is crucial and requires orientation of physicians to the significance of the study and the benefits to patients from participation in the study. The levels of approval for a study include: first, nursing support; second, physician approval; third, administrative support; and finally, human subjects' approval.

Experience has shown us not to expect much more than an introduction to the nursing unit to be involved. After these initial introductions, all attempts to proceed with the study come from the research team. Thus, the necessity of building good rapport with clinical nursing staff cannot be overemphasized (Pederson, 1980). It has become a habit, when a facility has granted access, to give at least one formal study orientation to the unit nursing personnel in order to introduce the research project and personnel. Several orientations may be necessary to cover all shifts. This introduction must be sensitive to the language barriers that may exist between the researcher and the staff. To avoid barriers, all research language should be left in the office (Todd & Gortner, 1982). During this time it is explained that all data will be collected without interrupting patient physical care and diagnostic procedures. It is understandable that nurse researchers are not always welcomed with open arms if staff anticipates an intrusion on nursing care delivery. Staff is assured that patient fatigue levels will be closely monitored and if necessary an interview will be postponed. Staff are also reminded that research assistants will not be providing nursing care. This information may come as good news or bad news, depending on the staff member.

Staff sensitivity to the research team may be decreased by frequent appearances on the unit, coffee with the head nurse and staff, establishing a relationship with the unit secretary, reading charts and checking Kardexes to see whether or not a potential subject exists. The more resistive the unit, the more frequently the research assistant must visit. The process of entrée is time-consuming and fatiguing but is rewarding when trust is established.

Whereas physician and Human Subjects Committee approval provide the formal green light to proceed, unfailing friendliness and occasional cookies have helped melt the hearts of the nursing staff.

Subject Accrual

When considering a particular facility for data collection, the researcher must discover the numbers of potential patients meeting the study criteria. For instance, one may want to study oncology patients with a colostomy. The researcher may check the census reports but few indicate the presence of a colostomy; most of the reports will indicate colorectal cancer, pelvic exenteration, or Crohn's disease. Moreover, patients may be found on a surgical floor, a gynecology floor, or medical floor. The search could be narrowed considerably by checking with the enterostomal therapist, if there is one, or with the operating room schedule. To be very precise, one could do a quick Kardex check for irrigation or bagging orders. No stone should be left unturned to accurately assess how many patients with a given diagnosis or surgery can be expected. The head nurse is an excellent resource for estimating the number of patients per week that fall within the study criteria. It is also possible to use the statistics from the same month in the previous year to estimate accurately. This information can be obtained from most medical record departments or cancer registries. One must also consider any potential change in surgeons or expected change in administration. Both may severely impact on the research study. Other authors have found, as we have, that when a population of patients is to be studied, suddenly there are no patients with that particular problem to be found (McHugh & Johnson, 1980). The problem of low subject accrual can be precluded somewhat by not drawing the criteria so tightly as to limit the study severely.

One researcher (Lewis, 1982) could only use those patients whose physicians diagnosed them as "terminally" ill. This requirement would severely limit potential subjects. In addition, one must be very creative in attempts at patient accrual. One researcher contacted the county medical examiner for names of the families of the deceased in order to complete a bereavement research study (Saunders, 1981). In fact, the medical examiner wrote a letter of condolence to the widows that introduced the researcher.

Obtaining a Consent

When approaching a patient for an informed consent, most research-oriented institutions and the federal government require that certain information be clearly presented to the patient. Patients have a right to know the study aims, the benefits, the risks, and compensation available if injury occurs, in addition to the time required to participate in the study. Furthermore, the subject must receive a copy of the Rights of Research Subjects (Table 10-7). The principal investigator and a witness must sign and date the consent.

There are various methods of approaching a patient for consent (Campbell, 1981). Sometimes a nurse from the unit may make an introduction or the research assistant may approach the patient "cold turkey." Before the actual approach, however, the research assistant has already read the medical record and, to the extent that it is possible, knows whether the patient meets the study criteria. For example, if the study is aimed at patients receiving radiation to the pelvis and disqualifies anyone with a previous history of pelvic radiation, the research assistant would have checked the history and physical and would not review the consent with an ineligible subject. This is not only a waste of time, but it is very embarrassing to offer participation in a study and then have to withdraw the invitation.

We have found that the most successful approaches are those made when the patient is comfortable, free of distractions (visitors, television, treatments), and is able to attend to the research assistants. If the patient is in an outpatient department waiting room with other patients within hearing, ask to speak to the patient privately, possibly after his or her appointment or treatment. Patient attention is limited if he or she may miss an appointment by not hearing her or his name called.

A positive attitude and a sensitivity to the feelings of the patients has helped accrue many subjects (Watson, 1985). The research assistants are taught to be persuasive without being pushy and to proclaim the benefits of participation to the patient. One education study in a radiation department (Padilla, 1983) had

TABLE 10-7. RIGHTS OF RESEARCH SUBJECTS

The rights below are the rights of every person who is asked to be in a research study. As an experimental subject, I have the following rights:
1. To be told what the study is trying to find out.
2. To be told what will happen to me and whether any of the procedures, drugs, or devices is different from what would be used in standard practice.
3. To be told about the frequent or important risks, side effects, or discomforts of the things that will happen to me for research purposes.
4. To be told if I can expect any benefit from participating and, if so, what the benefit might be.
5. To be told the other choices I have and how they may be better or worse than being in the study.
6. To be allowed to ask any questions concerning the study both before agreeing to be involved and during the course of the study.
7. To be told what sort of medical treatment is available if any complications arise.
8. To refuse to participate at all or to change my mind about participation after the study is started. This decision will not affect my right to receive the care I would recieve if I were not in the study.
9. To receive a copy of the signed and dated consent form.
10. To be free of pressure when considering whether I wish to agree to be in the study.

several patients simultaneously accrued and they kiddingly began calling each other by their study number instead of by name. This established a sense of camaraderie among those patients.

Maximizing Subject Retention

There are some basic techniques that will help the research team lose the minimum number of patients on the study. These have been described humorously (Atwood, 1980) but do reflect a potential problem for every researcher.

Some subjects will simply change their minds and not want to be involved in the study any longer. It is certainly the patient's option to withdraw his or her consent at any time. However, the urge to do something violent at the loss of a subject must be held in check. We attempt to find a reason for their change of heart, since it may have little to do with the project. We try to salvage the situation, but the researcher may have to be satisfied with little explanation. One culprit contributing to the attrition of subjects may be the volume of data requested. Because many of our studies contain weekly sets of questionnaires, we attempt to space the delivery of the instruments to reduce subject overload (Table 10–8). When patients begin to omit or lose tools, skip pages, or invent elaborate stories of how the neighbor's baby destroyed them, the problem may be data overload. To combat this, if the option is to lose the subject or decrease the data, we select the most essential questionnaires and delete the others. To minimize missing data because of skipped pages, we try to flip quickly through each tool while the patient is still present and ask the patient to fill in the missing information.

One must also consider the readability of the questionnaires in terms of language, size of type, and spacing on the page. Patients will quickly become frustrated if they cannot easily read the material (Topf, 1986). It is also impor-

TABLE 10-8. TIME SCHEDULE FOR INSTRUMENT ADMINISTRATION

WK 1	WK 2	WK 3	WK 4	WK 5
	Funct. age			
LOC				
POMS				POMS
Comply				
	Demographic			
	Support			Support
	Satisfaction			
Oral Assess	Oral Assess	Oral Assess	Oral Assess	Oral Assess
Nutrition			Nutrition	
I, II, III			I, II, III	
Anorexia		Anorexia		
Daily Record	Daily Record	Daily Record	Daily Record	Daily Record

tant to read the instructions on each questionnaire and, initially, to walk through each tool with the patient. This has helped remove any confusion in how to complete the forms.

One last word on overload. The nurse researcher may consider her- or himself in overload if a subject is lost because he expires and the nurse finds her- or himself angry with the patient. It has been our experience that patients do not intentionally do this.

Master Calendar

Organizing the data collection if there is more than one data collection period is always a challenge. The use of a master calendar helps relieve the stress of relying on memory and maximizes the efficient scheduling of appointments. A large-size month-by-month calendar with days boxed in 4- by 2½-inch spaces is useful. Each day is divided into segments for each data collection site. Each patient to be seen, the appointment time, the data collection week or tools to be used, and any other essential information is written on the calendar. Research assistant initials are penciled in next to the appropriate patient. This precludes any confusion about which assistant is seeing which patient. If the study has follow-up data to be obtained during outpatient appointments, it is important to arrange for outpatient computer access during off-hours so that the assistants can quickly find the patient's next appointment time without disturbing or interrupting any clinic personnel.

Preparing for Data Collection

Once the master calendar is set for a day (usually a few days before) all the tools that will be used for each patient are pulled, labeled with the appropriate subject numbers, and placed in a packet. When tools are sent home with a patient, a system for managing them is essential. In our studies, each subject has a bright-colored packet containing the questionnaires. The study patients are easily recognized by this packet, and if a new research assistant is seeing the subject, there is usually little difficulty in locating them. When the patient is seen, the completed tools are taken by the research assistant, and new tools added to the packet. At this time the completed tools are checked for any missing information so that they may be quickly completed by the patient. It is important that the data collection keep to a routine and be consistent across all subjects, regardless of the cast of characters. This routine avoids costly errors. Actually, it is most time- and cost-efficient to collect complete data the first time, whether from a patient or chart, to avoid duplication of the research assistant's effort.

Organizing Work Load

When more than one institution is used for data collection, organization of the work load is critical. If the study and patients allow, travel to facilities is planned when traffic is lightest. Try to stay clear of peak traffic hours and attempt to have an alternate route planned in the event of a traffic jam. Inevitably the research assistants will miss a subject, end up waiting for someone who is late, or have time between subjects. It is important to maximize this "down time." This is a good time to catch up on data coding, review the institution's schedule for possible subjects, check the patient's medical record for data needed, check in with the project director by telephone, do some public relations, or have lunch. Fortunately there are usually things that can be done to salvage time that would otherwise have been completely lost.

Coding, Verifying, and Filing

Once a subject has finished the study and the coding has been completed and checked by the research assistant, the data pack is given to the project director. It is important that the data be put in a designated order before they reach the project director. These "raw" data are checked thoroughly by the project director for completeness and accuracy. This involves scanning each record, remeasuring, recalculating, and generally scrutinizing the data for errors and omissions. All tools are then routed back to the appropriate research assistant to correct any errors that have occurred. The corrected record is then rechecked by the project director. This process, though laborious, has decreased our error rates to about 2 percent and makes for a very accurate data set.

There are various methods to use to file the raw data. For each subject, tools may be organized into separate folders by type or data collection period. Subject data may be organized by data collection site or by subject number (chronologically). Color coded tabs can also be used to identify subjects. For instance, subjects 001 to 030 may all have red tabs because they come from the same institution. Each subject will have three folders, and it is helpful to alternate the position of the tab after each subject number so the first three folders, all red with tab on the left, will read 001. The next subject, 002, will have three folders, all red and have a tab in the middle, and so on. This makes checking for the presence of all folders very simple.

Regardless of the method decided upon, a checklist is taped to the outside of each subject folder so that it is clear which pieces of data are to go in that particular folder. If the data are present in the folder, they are checked off. If they are missing, the letters "MD" are written next to the item on the checklist. All the subject's folders should be consistent, that is, the first folder for every subject should contain identical categories of data, and the same is true for the second and third folders as well. This simple system helps the project director to keep on top of large volumes of data.

Because the patient is entitled to and promised anonymity, all consent forms are filed separately from the subject's data. which is identified by a code number only. However, should it be necessary to retrieve information from a patient's chart, a confidential list of subject names and codes is kept in a master notebook by the project director. Furthermore, a master list of data required for each subject is checked off as tools are administered. This master list has been of immeasurable value in checking data already collected, as well as flagging all outstanding data (see Table 10-6).

Once data have been checked, they are ready for computer entry. All data entered in the computer are verified with the raw data (Barhyte & Bacon, 1985).

At this point errors in either the raw data or computerized data are found and corrected, further maximizing the accuracy of the data set.

BUDGET MANAGEMENT

Accuracy is the watchword of any research endeavor. It is required throughout the start-up activities, the data collection period, and the computer entry. Accuracy is also essential when the project budget is planned and the expenditures are monitored. It is always important to have the most current figures possible when reviewing the budget. Most institutional printouts run a minimum of 2 weeks behind in logging expenditures, and this may represent hundreds of dollars. It is essential for the principal investigator or project director to verify the accuracy of the summary expenditure reports soon after they are printed. These reports are usually subdivided into categories of expenses, simplifying the verification process. The report usually indicates monies granted, expenses to date, expenses in the current time period, and grant monies remaining.

The systematic expenditure review first compares the summary report with the salary distribution sheets to make certain the salary has been charged correctly and the total fringe amounts have been calculated appropriately. It is important to watch for errors such as employees being charged to the wrong grant account and incorrect fringe percentage calculations. Once the salary category is balanced, all miscellaneous charges must be reviewed including supplies, travel, consultant costs, and "other" categories. All these areas are cross-checked against all purchase requisitions, petty cash requests, and check requests. A keen eye must be kept for double charges as outstanding encumbrances that may take several months to show up on the expenditure reports. If discrepancies occur, the business office should be notified immediately by telephone and then by follow-up memo.

Any double charges or missed charges may take several weeks (if not months) to clear properly, giving a false balance and possibly a false sense of financial security. Eventually the day of reckoning will come and all the charges will be applied correctly. Scrutinizing the books carefully will avoid embarrassing and devastating overspending.

OTHER FACTORS

In addition to the information presented in this chapter, other factors contribute to the successful management of a research project. First, the satisfactory coordination of the research team is also affected by: number of participating institutions; autonomy of these institutions in relation to the project; number of investigators; autonomy of investigators; number of disciplines involved; and size of the research support staff. Second, efficient collection of data is also influenced by: number of sites and distance between sites at which data are collected; number of variables studied and research instruments used; times of the day or night during which data are collected; the variety of sources of data and complexity of the setting; number of subjects expected to participate; number and repetition of data collection episodes; and number and authority of subject gatekeepers. Third, successful management of the budget is also affected by the size of the budget; number and complexity of budget categories; involvement of subcontracts; and integration of project budget with other institutional or grant budgets.

REFERENCES

Atwood, J.R. (1980). Problems in doing research: How to maximize missing data and lose subjects. *Western Journal of Nursing Research, 2*, 425–427.

Barhyte, D.Y., & Bacon, L.D. (1985). Approaches to cleaning data sets: A technical comment. *Nursing Research, 34*, 62–64.

Bergstrom, N., Hansen, B.C., Grant, M., et al. (1984). Collaborative nursing research: Anatomy of a successful consortium. *Nursing Research, 33*, 20–25.

Campbell, H.M. (1981). Some common sense suggestions for nurses new at the research game. *The Canadian Nurse, 77*, 32–33.

Cronenwett, L.R. (1986). Access to research subjects. *Journal of Nursing Administration, 16*(2), 8–9.

Flaskerud, J.H., & Jamken, J.K. (1978). Research questions and answers. *Nursing Research, 27*, 375–376.

Kaempfer, S.H. (1982). A care orientation to clinical nursing research. *Oncology Nursing Forum, 9*, 36–38.

Lancaster, J. (1985). The perils and joys of collaborative research. *Nursing Outlook, 33*, 231–232, 238.

Lewis, F.M. (1982). Experienced personal control and quality of life in late-stage cancer patients. *Nursing Research, 31*, 113–119.

McHugh, N.G., & Johnson, J.E. (1980). Clinical nursing research beyond the methods books. *Nursing Outlook, 28*, 352–356.

Padilla, G.V. (1983). *Compliance strategies for cancer therapy* (Grant No CG 5R18CA-31164-01). Bethesda, MD: National Cancer Institute.

Padilla, G.V., & Grant, M.M. (1982). Quality assurance programme for nursing. *Journal of Advanced Nursing, 7*, 135–145.

Pederson, C.J., & Anderson, J.M. (1980). Factors that impact data collection from children. *Cancer Nursing, 3*, 439–444.

Rettig, F.M. (1980). Ideal attitudes of a nurse researcher. *AORN Journal, 32*(1), 62–64.

Saunders, J.M. (1981). A process of bereavement resolution: Uncoupled identity. *Western Journal of Nursing Research, 3*, 319–336.

Todd, A.H., & Gortner, S.R. (1982). Researchmanship removing obstacles to research in a clinical setting. *Western Journal of Nursing Research, 4*, 329–333.

Topf, M. (1986). Response sets in questionnaire research. *Nursing Research, 35*, 119–121.

Watson, P.G. (1985). Practical considerations for conducting nursing research. *Journal of Enterostomal Therapy, 12*, 182–185.

Cancer Nursing Studies

Saunders, J.M. (1981). A process of bereavement resolution: Uncoupled identity. *Western Journal of Nursing Research, 3*(4), 320–336.

LaMonica, E.L., Oberst, M.T., Madea, A.R., et al (1986). Development of a patient satisfaction scale. *Research in Nursing and Health, 9,* 43–50.

Lauer, P., Murphy, S.P., Powers, M.J. (1982). Learning needs of cancer patients: A comparison of nurse and patient perceptions. *Nursing Research, 31*(1), 11–16.

Lewis, F.M. (1982). Experienced personal control and quality of life in late-stage cancer patients. *Nursing Research, 31*(2), 113–119.

Padilla, G.F., Baker, V.E., Dolan, V. (1977). Interacting with dying patients. *Communicating Nursing Research, 8,* 101–114.

Dodd, M.J. (1984). Measuring informational intervention for chemotherapy knowledge and self-care behavior. *Research in Nursing and Health, 7,* 43–50.

Bishop, J.F., Olver, I.N., Wolf, M.M., et al (1984). Lorazepam: A randomized, double-blind, crossover study of a new antiemetic in patients receiving cytotoxic chemotherapy and prochlorperazine. *Journal of Clinical Oncology, 2*(6), 691–695.

The studies listed here are representative of different types of cancer nursing investigations and are used by the authors of the various chapters to illustrate theoretical or methodological points. Below are summaries of each of the articles with explanations of the editors' basis for their selection.

First is a qualitative study of the bereavement process in a group of young widows (Saunders, 1981). In this study, 12 widows were selected whose deceased husbands were between 30 and 39 years of age, Caucasian, Protestant, English-speaking, born in the United States, living within Los Angeles county, and died from causes that were natural ($n = 3$), accidental ($n = 3$), suicidal ($n = 3$), or homicidal ($n = 3$). In addition, 3 widows were chosen whose husbands were in the 40-to-49-year age range. This latter group was expected to provide natural contrast information. Widows were interviewed over a 13-month period. Although three response patterns were identified, the report focused on the process of developing an uncoupled identity. It was found that critical uncoupling experiences involved sorting the personal belongings of the deceased husband, deciding whether to wear the wedding ring, adjusting to changes in social interaction patterns, and dating.

Though the Saunders study is not about cancer patients or cancer nursing, it addresses an area of concern to oncology nurses, the bereavement experienced by family and significant others. The study reflects the richness of qualitative data as well as the difficulties in analyzing, summarizing, and interpreting the data. The study also provides a creative strategy for sampling subjects from a population that is very difficult to find and then approach.

Second is a series of three tool-development studies of a patient satisfaction scale (LaMonica et al, 1986). The scale included items revised from a previous instrument as well as new items, for a total of 50. A five-point response scale was used for each item. In study 1, 75 patients hospitalized for cancer treatment responded to the questionnaire. The criteria for retention were met by 42 items. These 42 items describing nurse behaviors (17 items were negatively worded) were then tested in study 2. Each of the 42 items had a seven-point Likert-type response scale ranging from strongly agree to strongly disagree. One hundred men and women undergoing cancer treatment responded to the 42-item scale. It was found that all items were skewed toward the positive end of the continuum. Based on the Risser study, items were grouped into three subscales: technical–professional, trusting relationship, and education relationship. Alpha coefficients for each of these subscales were satisfactorily high. Subscale intercorrelations indicated that the first two subscales overlapped. Study 3 tested the effects of an empathy training program on patient mood and satisfaction with nursing care with 710 patients hospitalized for cancer on two medical and two surgical units. An alpha coefficient of .95 for the total scale was obtained on 533 patients. High intercorrelations between subscales suggests that the 42-item scale is a unidimensional index. Factor analysis yielded three factors different from those conceptualized in the original tool: dissatisfaction (17 items), interpersonal support (13 items), and good impression (11 items). The first factor explained 73.6 percent of the variance, all three factors explained 93.7 percent of the variance. All three factors yielded alpha coefficients of .89 or better.

Tool development for the measurement of cancer nursing research variables is an important endeavor. In particular, measures of outcome variables are needed to evaluate the effects of nursing interventions. Tool development strategies also help to crystallize the dimensions of a concept. In the case of the LaMonica-Oberst Patient Satisfaction Scale, support was found for a three-factor but possibly unidimensional scale. In addition, results indicated that satisfaction and dissatisfaction may not be opposite anchors of the same continuum.

Third is a nonexperimental descriptive study comparing nurse and patient perceptions of the learning needs of cancer patients (Lauer, Murphy, & Powers,

1982). Of the 33 nurses from medical–surgical units who agreed to participate, 21 had less than 4 years of experience with cancer patients. The subject sample consisted of 27 cancer patients receiving chemotherapy or radiation therapy and readmitted at least once since initial diagnosis but not likely to die during the present hospitalization. The investigators developed a questionnaire of 36 items to evaluate nurse and patient perception of learning needs about nutrition, minimizing chemotherapy and radiation therapy side effects, recreational or work activities, relationships with significant others, understanding action of therapy, and dealing with feelings. Nurses ranked dealing with feelings as most problematic and as information patients want the most. Patients ranked minimizing side effects of therapy as most problematic and as information they want the most. The study showed the differences in nurse and patient perceptions of patient learning needs.

Descriptive studies are needed in cancer nursing to provide base line information about patient biopsychosocial responses to the cancer experience. Moreover, investigators may have to develop specific instruments for data collection in new areas. The Lauer, Murphy, and Powers study is important in cancer nursing because it provides some insight into factors that may contribute to patient compliance with treatment and self-care regimens. In general, patient education material is developed from the health-care provider's viewpoint about what is important for the patient and his or her family to know. This study reminds us that perceptions of need may be vastly different when nurses' views are compared with those of patients.

Fourth is an exploratory descriptive study with a correlational design that examined the association between experience of personal control over one's life and quality of life (Lewis, 1982). Fifty-seven cancer patients diagnosed as terminal by their physician responded to four questionnaires: the Rosenberg Self-Esteem Scale; the Health Locus of Control Scale; the Lewis, Firsich, and Parsell Anxiety Scale; and the Crumbaugh Purpose-in-Life Test. Subjects were preterminal (not actively dying), over 21, and on palliative medical management. The findings supported the hypothesis that experienced personal control over life was significantly related to quality of life as measured by self-esteem, anxiety, and purpose in life. Contrary to expectation, it was found that perceived personal control over health outcomes as measured by the health locus of control scale was an inconsistent predictor of quality of life.

Correlational studies of this type can contribute important information about the dynamics of cancer patient well-being. The issue of patient control underlies much of the interaction between nurses and patients. Health-provider values about what type and amount of control is appropriate for the patient or family to maintain, to give up, or to develop influence the assessment, care, and teaching of patients by oncology nurses. Lewis suggests that control may be positive or negative. For example, helping late-stage cancer patients to give up control over health may be an effective coping mechanism, while encouraging them to exercise control over other aspects of their life may contribute to their quality of life. Establishing the significance of relationships between patient variables is a necessary step to selecting and testing nursing interventions that are expected to have an impact on cancer patient outcomes.

Fifth is a report of three quasi-experimental studies of the effects of an in-hospital nursing education attitude-and-behavior-change program in improving nurse comfort and skill in caring for dying patients (Padilla, Baker, & Dolan, 1977). In study 1, three adult units were randomly assigned to an experimental ($n = 15$) and two control units ($n = 22$, $n = 17$). It was found that the experimental condition nurses who participated in the attitude-and-behavior-change program improved in their knowledge about the content of that program and in their communication skills. However, contrary to expectation, they felt less comfortable in situations with terminal patients. In study 2, ten nursing education instructors from ten different hospitals participated in the same attitude-and-behavior-change program. Their responses were compared to those of the staff nurses from the experimental condition in study 1. Pretest scores showed that the instructor group was more knowledgeable about the content of the program and more skillful in communication techniques than were the staff nurses. The posttest scores showed that the staff nurses improved slightly more in knowledge but did not surpass the instructors. Both groups improved in their communication skills, while the instructor group improved in their comfort scores. In study 3, the program was implemented across different institutional settings with different instructors for each institution to determine if the effects observed in study 1 could be replicated. Results from study 3 showed that, in general, the program contributed to greater knowledge about course content, increased comfort with dying patients, and improved communication skills with these patients, but it did not result in more positive patient affective states.

The three studies provide examples of the type of quasi-experimental program evaluation strategy that is feasible in clinical settings, where scientific control is difficult to implement. These studies illustrate the problems inherent in testing the impact of a program under conditions in which many factors cannot be controlled. Since both patient and nurse education programs are being developed in the area of oncology, it is important for nurses to test the effectiveness of these programs in bringing about desired knowledge, attitude, and behavior changes.

Sixth is an experimental factorial design that tested the impact of drug information and side-effect management information on chemotherapy knowledge, self-care behaviors, and general affective state (Dodd, 1984). The four-group design (drug information only, side-effect-management information only, both types of information, and no information) was carried out with 48 cancer patients, randomized 12 to a group. Subjects were over 18 and at least 2 weeks into an outpatient chemotherapy regimen. As predicted, patients who received drug information alone or with side-effect-management information had higher chemotherapy knowledge test scores than those who did not receive drug information. As expected, patients who performed the most self-care behaviors were those who received information about side-effect management. Contrary to expectation, the combination of both types of information did not result in more positive mood states.

This study by Dodd is important for two reasons. First, it represents the type of randomized, control-versus-intervention group study of the impact of nursing process on cancer patient outcomes that is the most valid strategy for establishing the scientific basis of oncology nursing practice. The study represents a logical progression from exploratory qualitative studies, to tool development and correlational descriptive studies, to randomized, control-versus-intervention group studies. Second, it demonstrates the importance of teaching in promoting positive outcomes for patients. Nursing is not alone in appreciating the critical role of patient information in fostering health-promoting behaviors. Other disciplines such as medicine, psychology, pharmacology, and so on, also recognize the importance of informational interventions. Because of the central role that nursing plays in patient care, nurses are in a unique position in the hospital, home, and community to test and implement information strategies. It is hoped that oncology nurses will proceed vigorously with such investigations either alone or in collaboration with other disciplines.

Seventh is a study of the effect of lorazepam on nausea and vomiting using an experimental, double-blind crossover study in which each subject was his or her own control (Bishop et al, 1984). This means that patients undergoing chemotherapy were randomized to one of six sequences of the antiemetic, lorazepam (L), and the placebo (P): LLP, LPL, LPP, PLL, or PLP. Drugs were packaged so that neither the patient nor the data collector knew what drug the patient was taking at any given time. Although 107 patients were randomized to one of these groups, only 80 could be evaluated because 14 did not complete both the lorazepam and placebo courses and 13 either died, were lost to treatment, or did not comply. It was found that lorazepam, when compared to placebo, significantly reduced patient experiences of the severity and duration of nausea, the severity of vomiting episodes, and increased sedation. Anxiety was reduced during the lorazepam versus placebo courses, but not significantly.

This study was selected for two reasons. First, it represents an important type of randomized experimental study, the double-blind, crossover clinical trial. The double-blind strategy is a classic approach to eliminating biased results. Neither the patient nor the data collector can be influenced by preconceptions of drug effectiveness. Applying this principle to the Dodd study would mean that the person collecting the data about patient knowledge of chemotherapy would not know whether the subject did or did not receive drug information. Such an approach would represent a single-blind study. Obviously, a double-blind study would not be possible, because the patient would know what type of information he or she received. The crossover procedure sets the subject as his or her own control so that the effects of the drug and placebo can be studied within the same patient. This strategy permits the investigator to evaluate the interaction of the intervention or placebo with the individual subject as well as the effect of the sequence of intervention and placebo. Second, this study exemplifies the typical clinical trial in which nurses are expected to participate as protocol nurses who carry out the study and as data collectors who measure and record patient responses. In any case, it is important for oncology nurses to appreciate the critical role that they play in the testing of drugs and other medical interventions.

These seven studies illustrate the diversity of scientific interests found among cancer nursing investigators. The studies also represent a variety of methodological approaches used to examine cancer nursing research questions. This diversity of interests and methods is critical to the development of the scientific foundation of cancer nursing practice in all its complexity.

Index